The Nutritionist's Kitchen

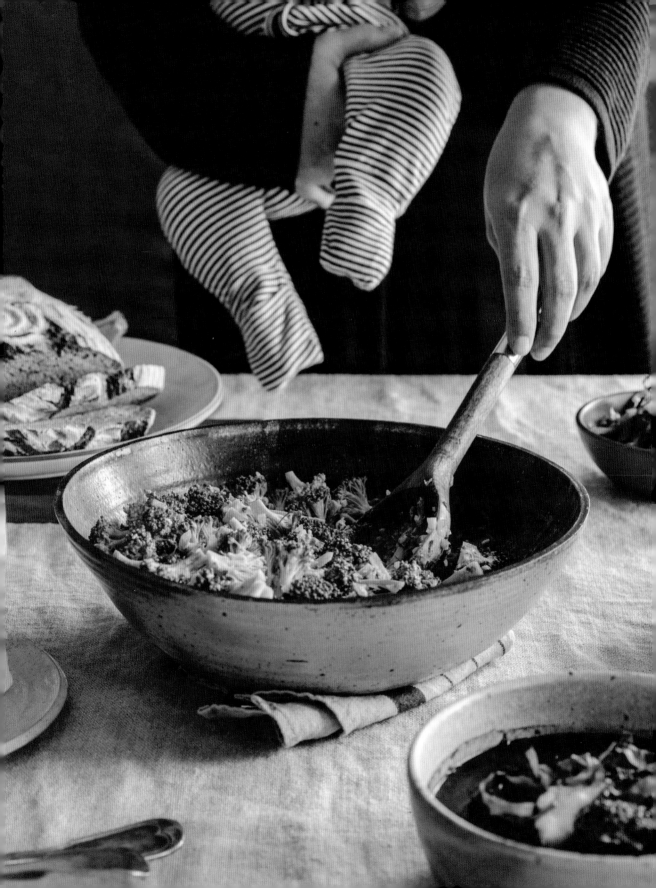

The Nutritionist's Kitchen

TRANSFORM YOUR DIET AND DISCOVER
THE HEALING POWER OF WHOLE FOODS

Carly Knowles, MS, RDN, LD

ROOST BOOKS

Roost Books
An imprint of Shambhala Publications, Inc.
4720 Walnut Street
Boulder, Colorado 80301
roostbooks.com

Cover design: Kara Plikaitis
Interior design: Laura Shaw Design

9 8 7 6 5 4 3 2

Printed in China

Library of Congress Cataloging-in-Publication Data

Names: Knowles, Carly, author.
Title: The nutritionist's kitchen: transform your diet and discover the healing power of whole foods / Carly Knowles.
Description: First Edition. | Boulder: Shambhala, [2020] | Includes bibliographical references and index.
Identifiers: LCCN 2019046796 | ISBN 9781611807172 (trade paperback)
Subjects: LCSH: Cooking (Natural foods) | Nutrition. | Health. | LCGFT: Cookbooks.
Classification: LCC TX741.K636 2020 | DDC 641.3/02—dc23
LC record available at https://lccn.loc.gov/2019046796

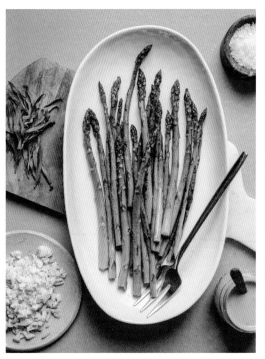
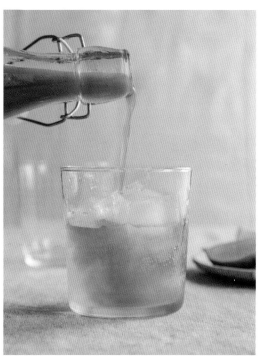
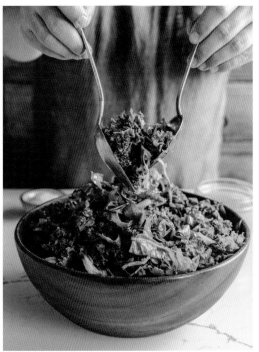
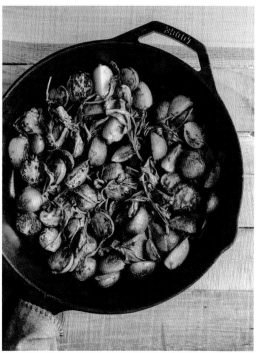

CONTENTS

PREFACE

I'VE ALWAYS HAD an insatiable hunger to travel and explore. When I was a small child, I would seldom stay in one place for long. When we dined out, which was often, I would leave the dinner table midway through the meal to meet and greet neighboring diners. When I was older, I traveled in more conventional ways—I lived with a host family in France in high school and managed to live and study abroad again in college. The instant I graduated, I packed my bags and embarked on my biggest adventure yet, to a very rural village in northern Peru. This time, I didn't buy a return ticket.

After a six-hour *camioneta* (small pickup truck) ride northeast from Piura into the desert and along the Andes, I was eventually dropped off in my new home—a town called San Francisco with a population of roughly two hundred. There was no running water in the village or electricity for miles, and the town's worn pay phone rarely, if ever, worked. It was remote, to say the least.

I worked with a U.S. nonprofit started by two Peace Corps volunteers, whose mission was to promote and sustain healthy behavioral change in rural and impoverished communities, specifically with youth. We collaborated with a local community organization to deliver basic health and hygiene education while promoting leadership skills, critical thinking, and healthy lifestyle activities. The days were long and hot, and the nights were too. The work was hard, personal time was hard to come by, and the local diet was extremely limited.

I found myself trying to get creative with meal planning, given our few ingredients. *How many ways could I rearrange these ingredients?* We had access to white rice, pig lard, white bread, plantains, bananas, beets, cilantro, lemongrass, chicken eggs, and on special occasions, dehydrated meat—typically including maggots from open-air storage. I was entertained at first trying to find new and tasty combinations. I once made a modified borscht (beet soup) that amused my host family for weeks—they would laugh at me daily and ask me why I would ever, for the love of God, drink pink soup!

Eventually, the novelty wore off, and I would crave fresh produce and protein. I didn't realize how much I relied on fresh food, especially produce, until then. I would stuff my backpack full of it when we took our monthly camioneta trips back to the city for meetings. Inevitably though, those foods didn't last long in the heat without refrigeration and would be gobbled up in a couple of days. The fresh fruit, local ceviche, heirloom corn, tricolor quinoa, guinea pig, spicy peppers, and abundance of colored potatoes Peru is known for were more than a thousand miles away in southern Peru.

At first, I could manage the limitations of this diet. It felt short term, and I was determined. After a few months, though, I didn't feel well. I slowed down a lot, gained weight, and felt worse in general. At the same time, I was trying to understand why many of the villagers had white spots growing on their eyes. Later, I discovered these were Bitot's spots and they were actually losing their eyesight due to a deficiency in vitamin A, a critical nutrient for vision, which is

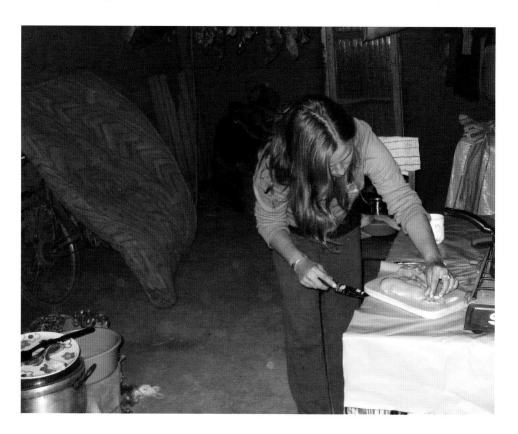

one of the leading preventable causes of blindness in developing nations. I also learned that vitamin A can easily be found in, among other foods, eggs, sweet potatoes, kale, spinach, pumpkin, whole cow's milk, and carrots.

As I learned more about nutrition and compared it to the local diet, I became more intrigued and fascinated and, frankly, concerned. Eating vitamin A–rich foods is enough to prevent blindness—whoa! Contrarily, not eating enough vitamin A–rich foods can lead to blindness. This was a profound moment for me. *Food really is medicine.* Before my epiphany, these were just fancy words I would read in fancy books and magazine articles or hear at new age juice shops in Portland, Oregon, where I'm from. My discovery also validated why I was feeling so dull and unhealthy.

A light turned on at that moment. This was the beginning of a new path for me. I could feel it in my bones. I knew right then and there, standing in my adobe room, that I had to learn as much as possible about optimizing your health with food and nutrition. I wanted to learn for those who aren't given the opportunity or don't know where to access reliable nutrition information. I wanted to study the foundation of nutrition, how we assimilate food, which foods provide which nutrients, how to prepare foods to maximize their nutrient content, and so much more I couldn't even fathom at the time. Specifically, I wanted to learn how to use food as medicine. I wanted to become a registered dietitian nutritionist.

Almost a year later, when I finally returned to the U.S., I applied and was accepted into the graduate program in nutrition at Bastyr University in Seattle, Washington. This is when I really started to understand the impact of nutrition and the incredible healing powers of food. Each meal, each snack, each sip of your favorite drink is another opportunity to nourish yourself. What you eat can actually prevent disease, help you function optimally, and even heal and restore your body. I was hooked.

INTRODUCTION

Food, people and the environment are synergistic. Separating
our food from the environment, or food from people, or the
environment from people encourages a lopsided view of the
world and forges lopsided solutions.

A-DAE ROMERO-BRIONES, FIRST NATIONS

AS WE LEARN more about the benefits of smaller sustainable food systems that
emphasize and strengthen a region's or community's overall well-being, we
also learn that local food systems promote the success of local food producers,
processors, distributors, consumers, and even food-disposal systems. This is
an alternative and more holistic approach to meeting our needs than the global
food system model that has dominated for so many years. Small and sustainable
food and agricultural initiatives actually have the potential to sustain a community's economic, social, and environmental health, as well as the quality of food
produced and the physical health of its people.

One way I believe we can make this shift and change our relationship with
our food and food system is by learning how to use food as medicine—a philosophy that honors self-care and puts quality, sustainable foods in the center.
We know that certain foods can actually prevent chronic disease and maintain
optimal health, so we can support ourselves and our families and maybe even
revolutionize our health care system by choosing to use our food as medicine.
But let's be honest, this is no simple task.

Changing our relationship with food can be complicated, and nutritional science is not straightforward. New and divisive research is published every year. There's conflicting information everywhere from "experts" in the field and many others too. There are countless new diets and health providers who swear they've found the magic pill. Even the food-as-medicine movement has become a righteous doctrine for some. It's a jungle out there, and I don't blame you for feeling overwhelmed at times. My goal as a registered dietitian nutritionist, and now as an author, is simply to streamline common principles of food as medicine and share the invaluable information I've learned throughout my formal and informal studies, while providing you with high-quality, nourishing, and flavorful recipes to help you bring this reality to life.

Since starting on this career path, I've had the great honor and privilege of working as a nutrition educator, registered dietitian nutritionist, and culinary instructor. I've met the most incredible people, patients, and participants on my journey and have learned so much about what it means to serve my community. Above all, I've learned more about nutrition and health directly from my patients than from any other source.

I've witnessed medical miracles with subtle diet changes, how impactful one cooking class can be for health outcomes, how transformational fresh food can be for a family, and the effect one bite of food can have for someone. *Food is powerful*. It can prevent disease, heal and restore the body, and sustain health over time. It can also heal and sustain a person's spirit. This philosophy is at the core of my work.

I hope this book will serve as a 101-style, foundational guide, providing you with trustworthy, evidence-based nutritional information, as well as a better understanding of your own intuitive medicine within. I share information to help you align yourself more closely with nature and the seasons while inspiring joy, promoting health, and creating magic in the kitchen with tasty, nutrient-dense recipes.

My intention was to create an approachable resource that feels like you're sitting with me or another registered dietitian nutritionist at home in your kitchen, sifting through nutrition information and finding what works best for you. Not everyone has access to a registered dietitian nutritionist, the time to see one, or the insurance to cover the costs, and that shouldn't be a barrier to learning this valuable health information.

I believe it all starts in the kitchen. Throughout this book, I emphasize the importance of cooking. The kitchen is not only the heart of a home but also a significant place to support and sustain your health and the health of your community. Research shows that those who cook and eat at home more often have better health and nutritional outcomes than those who eat out at full-service restaurants and fast-food chains. Research also shows that a lack of competency in food preparation is a primary barrier to making healthy food. Those who start cooking as teens and young adults (ages eighteen through twenty-three) have better long-term, nutrition-related outcomes, such as more frequent vegetable consumption and less frequent fast-food consumption.

I've organized the recipes by seasons: spring, summer, autumn, and winter. I hope they inspire you to cook and eat more in rhythm with nature, giving yourself the opportunity to live in sync with your regional climate while also supporting your local food economy and environment. Plus, food that's in season—such as delicate pea tendrils in the spring or sun-ripened tomatoes in the summer—undeniably has more flavor.

You'll find vegetarian and vegan recipes in this cookbook mixed in with recipes that include dairy, meat, poultry, and seafood. Truly, there's something for everyone. The common thread between the recipes is the celebration of fresh, minimally processed, whole food ingredients.

Please refer to these abbreviations at the top of each recipe:

GF	Gluten Free	**Ve**	Vegan
DF	Dairy Free	**RT**	Requires Time
V	Vegetarian		

What Is a Registered Dietitian Nutritionist?

A registered dietitian (RD) or registered dietitian nutritionist (RDN) is a nationally certified nutrition expert who has a minimum of a bachelor's degree in nutrition and dietetics from an accredited college or university. These individuals are required to complete an accredited supervised six- to twelve-month internship and also pass a national certified exam before practicing. By the year 2024, all registered dietitian nutritionists will be required to have a minimum of a master's degree.

Registered dietitian nutritionists work with insurance companies to bill reimbursable hours for their patients in hospitals, medical clinics, and private practice. They are familiar with a variety of subjects, including but not limited to food and nutrition sciences, food service systems management, business, economics, computer science, culinary arts, sociology, biochemistry, physiology, microbiology, anatomy, and chemistry.

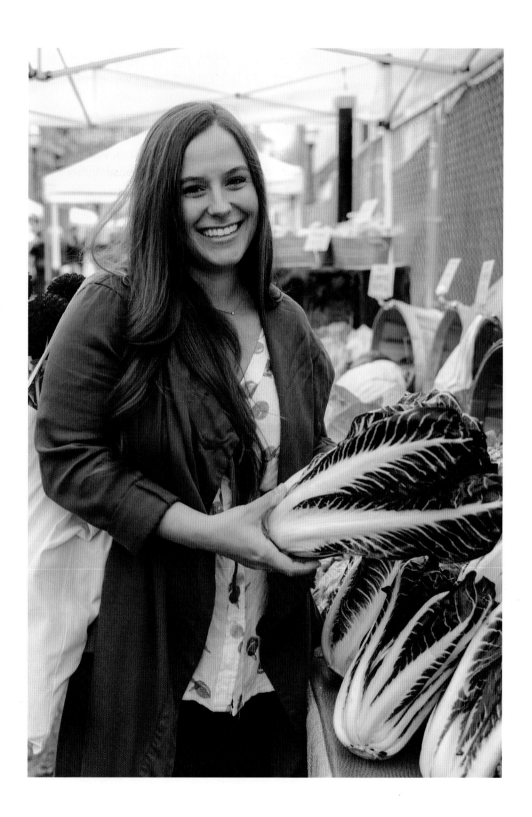

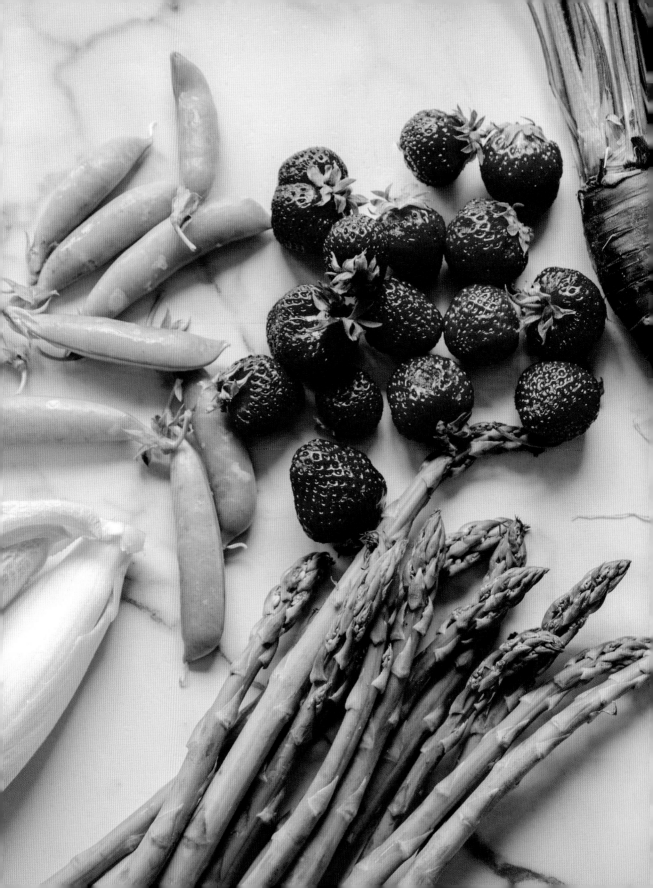

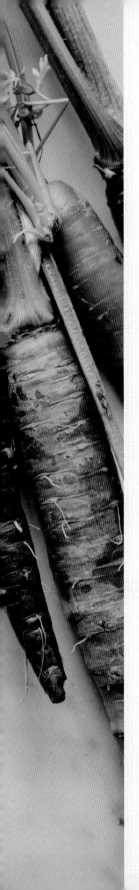

PART ONE

YOUR GUIDE TO USING WHOLE FOODS AS MEDICINE

1
THE PRINCIPLES

The doctor of the future will give no medicine
but will instruct his patient in the care of the
human frame, in diet and in the cause and
prevention of diseases.

THOMAS EDISON

FOOD IS ONE of the most powerful and effective forms of medicine. It's more than just fuel. It contains a wide variety of vitamins, minerals, phytonutrients, bioactive compounds, antioxidants, and more, all of which can prevent disease, heal and restore the body, and maintain long-term health and optimal function. Food can also bring you joy and inspire human connection.

Possibly the most effective way to use food, though, is for the prevention of disease. Now, more than ever before, we have access to scientific research that shows the impact of healthy eating patterns on disease. For example, we know that eating a plant-based diet can significantly reduce your risk for certain health conditions, including coronary artery disease or heart disease, certain types of cancer, obesity, and type 2 diabetes. A diet rich in vegetables, fruits, legumes, whole grains, soy products, nuts, and seeds can reduce cholesterol levels and help to control blood glucose levels. Adopting healthy diet and lifestyle practices before and during pregnancy can also prevent significant risks, including birth defects, suboptimal fetal development, and chronic health problems in both mother and child. The list goes on and on.

But food can do more than just prevent disease. It can also help to heal and restore the body after medical issues or diseases have already set in. For example, we know that regulating carbohydrate intake at mealtimes is therapeutic for blood sugar management for type 2 diabetes. And including a source of vitamin C with iron-rich foods can help to increase the absorption of iron in those with iron deficiency anemia.

Many medical conditions and diagnoses actually have a specific evidence-based therapeutic diet and nutritional recommendations called medical nutrition therapy (MNT), which are delivered by a registered dietitian nutritionist or physician. MNT is the gold standard for nutrition care management and includes nutritional diagnosis, therapy, and counseling services. All MNT recommendations have been thoroughly studied and are applied and upheld internationally in the medical community.

And there's more! An emerging subject within nutritional sciences, and one of my favorite topics in the field, is the study of nutrigenomics, or the nutritional factors of the human genome—the genetic material of which we're made. Because of nutrigenomic research, we now know, for example, that various antioxidants and phytochemicals found in our food enhances DNA repair and reduces oxidative damage, which recent research has suggested may even compensate for inherited genetic defects. Researchers are also finding that nutritional imbalances can increase DNA or genome damage and that maintaining a nutrient-dense, balanced diet may help to prevent this damage.

Perhaps, though, the real purpose of why we eat cannot be intellectualized or made into science, but rather only felt in spirit. I bet you can recollect at least one fond memory, if not many, where food was the centerpiece—those moments when food nourished your soul. Gathering for communal meals, breaking bread, and strengthening the human bond have been documented as common practices dating over three hundred thousand years. Preparing and sharing food not only connects us to others and brings us great satisfaction and joy, but it can also help us to develop food agency (individual, technical cooking and food provisioning skills considering cognitive capacities and social and cultural support and barriers). And in a time when poverty, food insecurity (lack of consistent access to enough food for a healthy and active life), and chronic disease plague populations, people's belief in the ability to feed and nourish themselves and their families is paramount. Researchers are also finding that sharing the same food, whatever it may be, and not just sharing a table may actually play a role in establishing trust and cooperation, as well as provide a feeling of closeness within a group of people.

What Qualifies Food as Medicine?

The question I get asked the most as a registered dietitian nutritionist is, "What is the ideal diet?" My answer is simple—there is none. We all need something different. We need different nutrients for different reasons at different life stages. So, where do you start then? Simply put, at the end of the day, I recommend that everyone starts with real food comprising whole, unprocessed, and unrefined ingredients. Outside of your personal dietary needs, there are some basic practices you can adopt to transform your food into medicine.

In the following sections, I've highlighted the pillars of food as medicine using a collection of evidence-based nutrition and research as well as intuitive insight I've gleaned along the way.

1. Choice and Awareness

In order to transform your food into medicine, you must first *see* your food as medicine. You have to make a conscious choice and commitment to yourself. This is the first step. Bring awareness and curiosity to your plate or bowl. Instead of relegating medicine to pharmaceuticals, make the choice to eat food with life-giving energy versus food that depletes you of that energy. Are you ready to see your food in this way? Do you really think it can prevent disease and/or help you heal? Once you take this first step, you'll never look back.

2. Whole Foods

Eat food that exists in nature. The definition of whole foods is just that—real food that you can picture living and growing in its whole form in nature before it makes its way to your grocery store or farmer's market. Both plants and animals can be whole foods. Salmon, blueberries, and rice are examples of whole foods. You can visualize where they come from and imagine how they existed in nature before they were caught, picked, or cultivated. Whole foods can also include minimally processed foods, such as those that have been pickled, ground, milled, or baked. Whole grain flour, nut butter, fruit jam, pickled carrots, and cooked rolled oats all qualify as whole foods since they are only minimally processed into their new form.

Another way to highlight whole foods is to choose food that has history. Food that has been around for a long time (at least one hundred years) is here to stay. Trendy food may come and go, but real food is timeless. Grains, fish, fruit—these are all ancient whole foods that date back thousands of years. Bread, pickles, noodles—these are tried-and-true and aren't going anywhere any time soon—and thank goodness! The benefits of eating and thinking of food in this way is that you're not using yourself as an experiment. New age, synthetic foods include ingredients and processes that are so new we don't yet understand their long-term impacts on our health. Some may pan out to be OK, and others will not (think trans fats, artificial sweeteners, food preservatives, and so on). Keep yourself safe and sane, and choose food that has history.

WWGD (What Would Grandma Do)?

This is a saying that my husband and I came up with when we were traveling in Spain. We were blown away by the beautiful open-air markets, and although they were often filled with tourists like us, we were amazed to see so many locals shopping there too. We remember specifically at one of the larger markets, this one local, elderly woman with her rolling basket and her bright, mission-driven eyes. She pushed us aside and made her presence known at the olive booth. Shortly after she left, the purveyor told us that she had been coming to his family's stall weekly for over forty years. We watched her as she rolled away and made her rounds, collecting her weekly bounty.

We sat with our *pintxos* (snacks) outside the market and found ourselves talking more about this tenacious woman. What truly amazed us was the fact that she most likely had to travel to multiple markets every week to get all of her ingredients since each market sells limited food groups. She was also most likely limited to seasonal and traditional foods since that's what most markets carry, and she could buy only as much food as would fit in her rolling basket.

We compared this experience to ours at home in the States, where most of us can get our groceries and all other necessary things at one large supermarket with rows and rows of convenience items, most of which we don't need. Whether by choice, necessity, ritual, or convenience, this woman traveled by foot, weekly, to multiple markets for her foraged finds—and she got not only her goods but also her exercise.

We decided to call her Grandma, and we vowed then and there to ask ourselves more often, "What would Grandma do?" Would she shop at a supermarket chain, or would she walk from one local community market to another collecting her goods? Would she experiment with new manufactured foods or opt for trusted, traditional, whole foods? Would she choose fast food, or would she cook herself a homemade meal? Would Grandma use a new age kitchen gadget to make dinner in a hurry, or would she use her favorite fifty-year-old Dutch oven with worn handles and spend the day cooking? Now, I know we're romanticizing the situation a bit (OK, a lot!), and there are many types of grandmas out there, but she really did inspire us to slow down and get back to basics in both how we shop and cook and, frankly, how we interact with the world. So when I talk about eating food with history, what I'm really asking you is, "What would Grandma do?"

3. Organic Foods

Prioritizing organic foods, both plant and animal, can benefit your health. However, it's not necessary to eat organic all the time. If you have this luxury, you're doing great! Unfortunately, though, organic foods typically (but not always) cost more and may not be easily accessible where you live.

A QUICK REVIEW OF ORGANIC FARMING

Organic farming for both plants and animals, according to U.S. law, cannot include synthetic fertilizers, sewage, most synthetic pesticides, genetically modified organisms (GMOs), irradiation, and antibiotics or growth hormones for animals. Organic farming promotes soil and water quality, reduces pollution, is self-sustaining, provides healthy and safe environments for animals (including pasture-feeding and organic feed), and supports natural behavior in animals.

On average, shoppers can save 89 percent of the total cost of organic foods when purchasing organic beans, grains, and nuts in bulk compared to their packaged counterparts. Buying in bulk also reduces the negative environmental impact from unnecessary product packaging. Win-win!

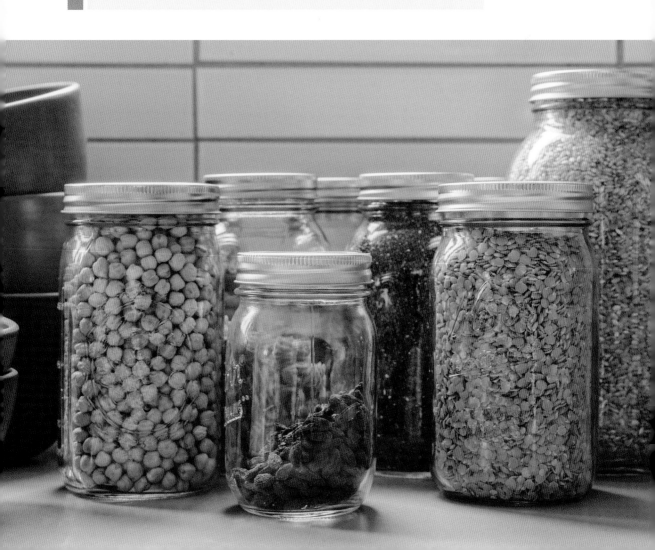

What Are GMOs, and Do I Need to Worry about Them?

Genetically modified organisms or genetically engineered (GE) foods are plants, bacteria, viruses, fungi, and animals whose genetic code has been altered in some way in a laboratory. This process creates a new and artificial genetic code that cannot be found in nature. Today, most genetic engineering is used to develop newer and stronger herbicides and insecticides to produce higher crop yields for farming (mostly soy, corn, sugar beets, and canola), but a growing number of GMOs can be found in our food system in cow, chicken, and salmon production.

Since the majority of European countries banned GMO foods more than twenty years ago, the need for chemicals and pesticides in local farming has actually been reduced by about 65 percent.

I recommend avoiding GMOs whenever possible, especially those exposed to glyphosate, a popular herbicide, because preliminary research shows an increased risk for food allergies and even cancer when this chemical is consumed. Although more large-scale studies need to be conducted before we can confirm these findings, there's no harm in avoiding GMOs. Look for the Non-GMO Project Verified label on packaging to ensure that a food product is composed of GMO-free ingredients.

Also, food for thought: GMOs are mostly used in agricultural farming to increase a crop's growing season, decrease its harvest time, and improve its stamina in various growing conditions. One could argue that these are natural limitations placed on us by the environment, all of which encourage us to live within our local climate and season, the benefits of which have been shown, time after time, to support our health and longevity, pocketbooks, and local economy.

 Look for the U.S. Department of Agriculture (USDA) organic label when buying organic foods. This label ensures that the ingredients and materials used to grow or raise that food are at least 95 percent organic. It also ensures that any nonorganic products used are commercially unavailable otherwise.

As the popularity of organic food and farming increases, we hope to learn more about the compositional differences between organic and conventional foods. Multiple studies conducted (mostly in the past decade) show a small but promising difference between the nutrient content in some conventional and organic foods. In one study, organic fruits and vegetables were shown to have a lower concentration of nitrates and higher vitamin and mineral content, as well as a higher percentage of bioactive compounds (naturally existing chemicals found mostly in plants that promote good health). In another study, organic meat and dairy were shown to have more omega-3 fatty acids, or healthy fats, than their conventional counterparts and a more beneficial ratio of omega-3 to omega-6 fatty acids.

In other studies of organic versus nonorganic grains, the organic variety was shown to contain less cadmium (a toxic chemical found in soil and absorbed by plants), which may be due to organic farming practices. Finally, organically grown foods are shown to have lower levels of pesticide residue than conventionally grown foods, which may be related to the strict regulations against pesticide use in organic farming.

Since the subject of organic versus nonorganic is complex, and scientific opinion is divided, the following list can act as a guide or starting place for you when considering each food group.

FRUITS AND VEGETABLES

There's some give-and-take when considering which fruits and vegetables to buy organic versus nonorganic or conventional. My recommendation is to prioritize the Dirty Dozen when buying organic produce. The Environmental Working Group (EWG) has created the "Shopper's Guide to Pesticides in Produce" that lists the twelve fruits and vegetables with the highest exposure to pesticides, fertilizers, and toxic chemicals. The EWG also highlights the fifteen fruits and vegetables with the least exposure to harmful toxins, called the Clean Fifteen. These lists are updated every year based on new data, so it's important that you check back annually. You can order a hard copy version of the guide or download the EWG's free and convenient app for your phone to use while grocery shopping. I can't recommend this resource strongly enough.

OTHER THINGS TO CONSIDER WHEN BUYING ORGANIC FRUITS AND VEGETABLES

- **Buy seasonal produce.** Fruits and vegetables naturally grow with less effort and human intervention when they're cultivated and harvested in season rather than forced to grow out of season with the use of fertilizers and pesticides.

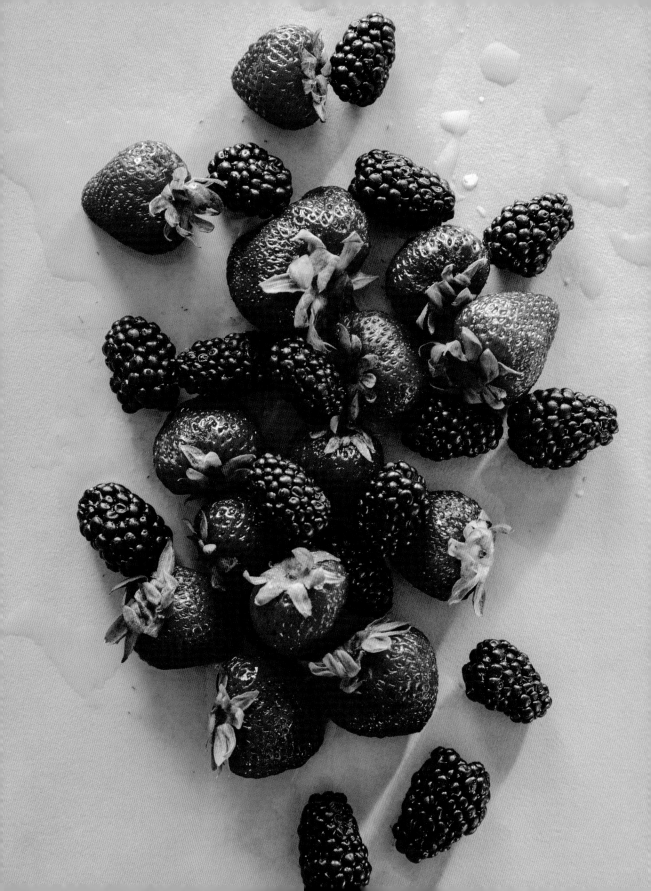

- **Look for produce with thick peels and casings.** Produce with thicker peels or casings, such as onions, melons, and kiwis, are generally better protected from chemical exposure than those with tender exteriors. There are exceptions to this rule, however. Peeling the outer layers of your produce can help to reduce chemical toxins but may compromise the nutrient quality.

- **Look for stickers on your produce with a price look-up (PLU) code that starts with the number nine.** All organic/non-GMO fruits and vegetables sold in the U.S. will have this code.

- **Wash your fruits and vegetables well.** Thoroughly washing and scrubbing your produce can reduce harmful bacteria and remove some, but not all, pesticide residue. Consider buying a produce scrub brush.

- **Eat a variety of fruits and vegetables.** Eating different types of produce from various sources reduces your risk of exposure to any one specific chemical toxin. You will also vary your nutrient intake by eating a diverse array of foods from different places.

BEANS AND LEGUMES

There's little evidence to support claims that organic beans or legumes are better for you or contain fewer toxins. With the exception of soybeans, this is a category or food group where you can roam in the nonorganic section without as much worry. Conventional beans and legumes are a fine choice. My recommendation and first choice is to purchase dried beans, whenever possible, from a trustworthy source. If buying canned beans, make sure you read the label. Oftentimes, there are more additives in your canned food than you may think.

Soybeans, however, vary slightly from other beans and legumes. Buy organic soy whenever possible. For myself and my family, this is a must, because 90 percent of all the soybeans produced in the U.S. are genetically modified and they have one of the highest percentages of contamination by toxic pesticides in our food that has been thoroughly studied. Soybeans are also one of the most highly processed foods both here and internationally, leading to many questionable and suboptimal "edible" by-products that spill over into our grocery stores and onto our plates as soy isolates, hydrolyzed soy protein, and other man-made soy foods. There has been limited research on the long-term health implications of these by-products and, thus, I recommend limiting or avoiding them for now.

EGGS, DAIRY, MEAT, AND POULTRY

With these foods, I definitely recommend buying organic. Although there is limited research on whether they actually contain fewer chemical toxins, they have been shown to contain more nutrients. Specifically, organic dairy and meat contain an average of 50 percent more omega-3 fatty acids compared to the conventional versions. Eating organic eggs, dairy, meat, and poultry may also help to reduce the development of antibiotic resistance in humans, since organically raised animals never come in contact with antibiotics.

Aside from the nutritional benefits, I recommend organic eggs, dairy, meat, and poultry due to the sad and intolerable treatment of animals on factory farms, which accounts for 99 percent of all farm animals in the U.S., as well as the devastating environmental consequences of large industrial farming. Animals are overcrowded and confined to small cages indoors with poor air quality and unnatural light. They're unable to engage in natural behaviors, are fed unnatural diets to increase muscle and fat stores, and are often given growth hormones and are physically altered in an effort to produce higher yields. The unsanitary conditions and poor treatment lead to infections and diseases that require antibiotics and various other medications to control, which studies have found are present in the animals' meat. As mentioned previously, organic farming standards exclude genetic engineering, ionizing radiation, and sewage sludge feed.

 CERTIFIED HUMANE. Another label to look for when considering animal welfare is the Certified Humane Raised and Handled label. This ensures transparency and accountability from farmers (organic or conventional) who produce products from farm animals. It certifies that the animals were humanely raised and slaughtered according to regulated care standards upheld by veterinarians, scientists, and

Animals raised in concentrated animal feeding operations (CAFOs) or factory farms are fed mostly grains, oils, ground animal parts (from dead, dying, diseased, and disabled animals), animal waste, antibiotics and other drugs, and plastics.

third-party inspectors through annual audits. Animals are never confined to battery cages, gestation crates, or tie stalls. They receive nutritious diets without antibiotics or growth hormones. They have access to shelter and resting areas, as well as space to support natural behaviors.

 GRASSFED. Organic eggs, dairy, meat, and poultry aren't always easy to find, and smaller farms can't always afford the expensive organic certification processes, even when they're practicing organic farming. An alternative, although not the same thing, is to purchase 100 percent grassfed or pasture-raised meat from a reputable local farm, farmer's market, or cooperative where you can rely on quality practices. Look for the American Grassfed Association's certification logo, which means that the animals ate a natural foraged diet all their lives, were raised on a pasture and not indoors or in a confined space, and were never treated with hormones or antibiotics. Grassfed or pasture farming also promotes a cleaner environment and has been shown to reduce greenhouse gas emissions by reducing atmospheric carbon dioxide with larger green spaces.

Finally, research shows that grassfed beef, milk, milk-derived products such as yogurt and cheese, and poultry are more nutritionally dense than their conventional counterparts—similar to organic dairy, meat, and poultry. Mostly, the fat quality of grassfed foods is better. Specifically, they contain more vitamin A and E, higher amounts of omega-3 fatty acids, higher-quality saturated fat, a better omega-3/omega-6 fatty ratio, and increased amounts of conjugated linoleic acid (CLA). The latter is a beneficial fat that has been shown to reduce inflammation, support immune function, improve bone mass and blood sugar regulation, and reduce body fat.

> One pound of factory farmed or feedlot beef produces about 26 pounds of carbon dioxide emissions. Skipping one serving of (factory farmed) beef one day a week for one year saves the emissions equivalent of driving a car 348 miles. Meatless Mondays, anyone?

NUTS

My recommendation here is to buy organic shelled nuts or conventional whole nuts with their shells intact. Conventional nuts are regularly sprayed with pesticides and fungicides before, and sometimes even after, they're shelled, which has been shown to be toxic to both humans and animals. Buying organic nuts, shelled or not, ensures little to no chemical exposure.

Because nuts contain high amounts of fats and oils, they more readily absorb chemical toxins (which are fat-soluble) used in the growing and harvesting process. Buying conventional nuts with their shells intact can help to lower chemical exposure given that the shell helps to protect the edible meat inside. Finding nuts that include their shells can be challenging, though, unless you buy directly from a farm or at a farmer's market. Organic shelled and raw nuts are a great alternative.

SEEDS

There's not a lot of evidence-based nutrition information available comparing organic to nonorganic seeds. Most seed research focuses on the study of organic seeds in regard to farming and food production rather than directly as a food source. Given the nature of most seeds as a healthy fat source, apply many of the same guidelines to seeds as you do to nuts. Buy conventional or nonorganic seeds if they come with a shell or hull or, to err on the side of caution, buy organic shelled and hulled seeds.

In general, when considering whether to buy organic or nonorganic foods that don't have a lot of available research—or all foods, for that matter—consider first if it's a big agricultural commodity, like sunflower seeds, which are one of the five largest oilseed crops in the world. If it's popular, then it's likely to be exposed to more fertilizers, pesticides, and other chemicals for higher and faster yields in a competitive market.

WHOLE GRAINS

I recommend buying organic barley, corn, sorghum, oats, rice, rye, and wheat in any form (such as whole, flour, or syrup), as these grains are some of the top U.S. agricultural commodities and profitable exports. Conventional forms are likely laden with chemicals and toxins used to increase production and yield.

Nutritionally, organic wheat has been shown to contain significantly more zinc than conventionally grown wheat, which is especially beneficial in developing countries and regions of the world where zinc deficiency is more common. Given, though, that only 4 percent of all food produced in the U.S.

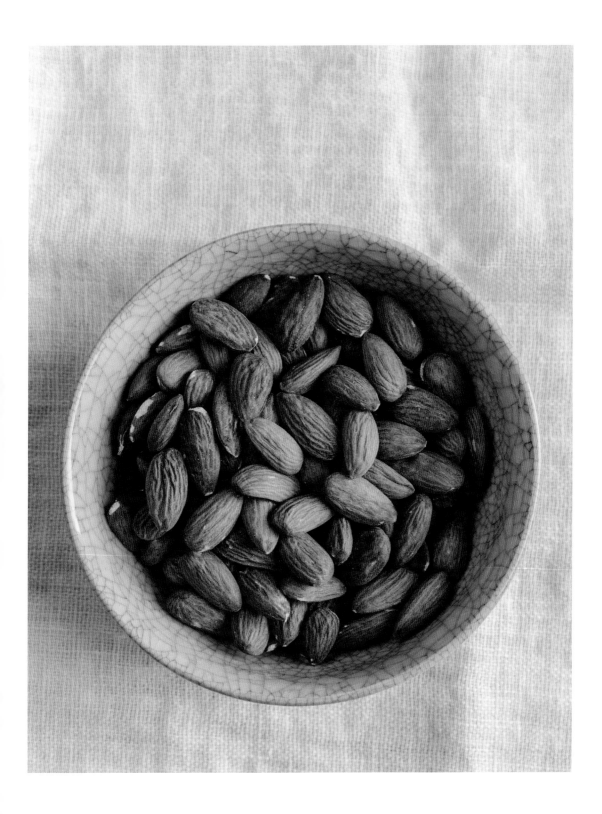

is certified organic, we lack studies at this time to determine any further health benefits of organic grains versus conventional ones.

4. Diverse Nutrient Profile or Nutrient Density

Nutrient density is a measure or concentration of nutrients in a certain amount of food or the amount of calories in that food. To simplify this concept, think of two different foods side by side and ask yourself which one has more nutrients bite for bite. This is an example of nutrient density. A bite of breakfast porridge, such as Buckwheat Breakfast Porridge with Cranberry Chia Compote (page 119), made from whole grains, seeds, and berries has more nutrient density than a bite of colorful, sugary breakfast cereal.

Choose food that has a diverse nutrient profile or is naturally nutrient dense. Food with a diverse nutrient profile contains beneficial vitamins and minerals with very little saturated fat, added sugar, sodium, or refined starches. Other examples include beans, eggs, fruits, seafood, vegetables, and whole grains. By focusing on a whole foods diet, you'll find that it's not very hard to eat nutrient-dense foods.

A tool I use to help people identify nutrient-dense foods is to promote rainbow-colored meals and snacks. If your plate of food is colorful like a rainbow, it most likely contains a diverse array of nutrients. Naturally colorful foods typically indicate a high vitamin, mineral, and phytonutrient content, which is essential for health. Eating a colorful diet can help you get a wider variety of beneficial nutrients. Read more about rainbow food in Chapter 2 (page 39).

The Power of Two

This is something I made up to help my patients more easily recognize nutrient-dense foods. If a food item includes a notable amount of at least two major macronutrients (protein, fats, carbohydrates) or micronutrients (vitamins, minerals), you're eating a food with lots of nutrients. Almond butter, for example, is loaded with healthy fats and protein, as well fiber, vitamin E, and biotin (more than two nutrients!), so you confidently know you're eating a nutrient-dense food. Lentils contain a substantial amount of protein, iron, folate, fiber, and many other vitamins and minerals (again, more than two), so you know they're full of nutrients. For comparison, donuts, although delicious, don't contain much other than carbohydrates, saturated fat, and sugar.

5. Unprocessed/Minimally Processed and Unrefined

Do your best to get your daily nutritional intake from unprocessed or minimally processed and unrefined foods. Added sugar, sodium, and trans fats are some of the biggest hazards of processed foods. Added sugar is often used in low-fat or nonfat products to improve the taste and consistency and is linked to heart disease, diabetes, unintentional weight gain, inflammation, fatty liver disease, and high blood pressure. Sodium is used mostly to enhance flavor and act as a preservative. It's found in almost every box, bottle, and can of highly processed food and can lead to high blood pressure, heart attacks, and strokes. Trans fats, or partially hydrogenated oils, provide body and texture to foods and keep them shelf-stable; unfortunately, they also increase levels of low-density lipoprotein (LDL) cholesterol (also called bad cholesterol) and have been widely linked to heart disease and even death. Fortunately, as of June 2018, the majority of trans fats were banned from the U.S. food supply, although their negative impact will be seen for decades to come. The Food and Drug Administration (FDA) extended the date for implementation of the ban to January 2020 for a small group of manufacturers to allow for an "orderly transition." An even smaller group of manufacturers is waiting until January 2021. These uses include as a solvent or carrier for flavoring agents, flavor enhancers, and coloring agents in processed foods, as well as a pan release agent for processed baked goods.

Highly processed foods generally contain a long list of ingredients, many of which are man-made (and hard to pronounce). As a rule of thumb, if your ingredient list includes ten or more ingredients, check the label and consider another available brand with fewer ingredients or see if you can make a simpler version at home instead. Preservatives, food coloring, artificial flavorings, chemical sweeteners, and other foreign ingredients are often included in highly processed foods and have been linked to diabetes, hypertension, and unintentional weight gain.

The term *refined* indicates a process that typically refers to grains and sugar but can also be applied to cooking oils. Grains are processed and stripped of most of their vitamins and minerals, as well as fiber, to create a "better" tasting food with a finer texture that's more shelf stable. This is the process of turning a whole grain into a refined grain. Refined sugars include white table sugar, high-fructose corn syrup, dextrose, and many other sweeteners that are the primary cause of high caloric intake, according to the *American Journal of Preventive Medicine*. This can lead to diabetes, obesity, and other serious health problems. Refined oils are filtered, heat treated, and mixed with

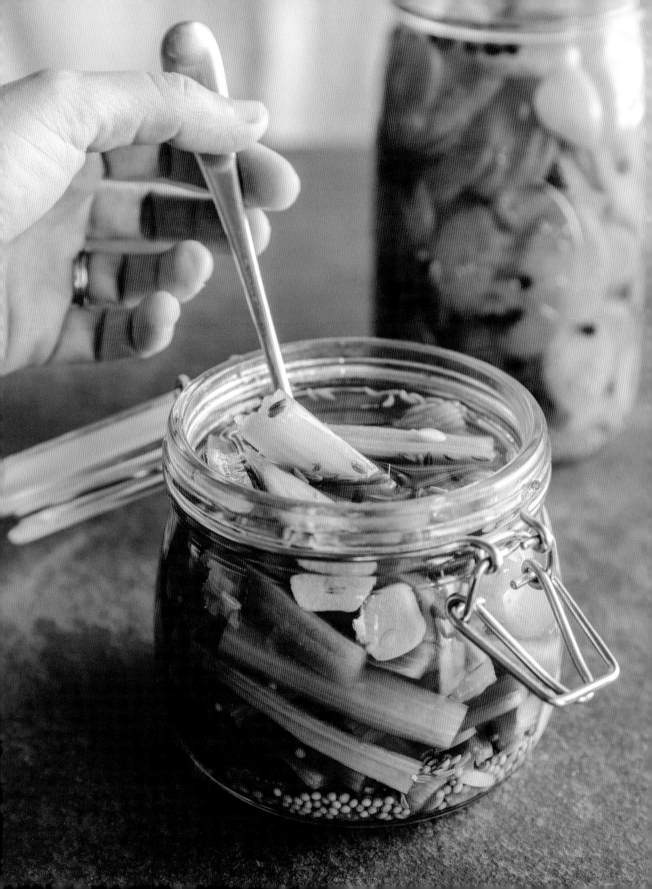

chemicals to create tasteless, more shelf-stable oils. Additionally, refined oils often include genetically modified ingredients and more free radicals, which have also been shown to be extremely hazardous to our health. Make sure to read labels and choose "unrefined" foods whenever possible.

This may surprise you, but some processed foods are actually supportive of a healthy diet and lifestyle. Yes, you read that right. There are plenty of processed food items I love and even recommend to my patients, including coconut milk, pickles, canned tomatoes, and almond flour. Minimally processed foods are totally OK and are oftentimes a great source of beneficial nutrients. Cutting, blending, milling, pickling, and so on are all basic forms of processing that don't include hidden ingredients or harmful additives while keeping the ingredient list fairly short. See the difference?

6. Simple, Quality Ingredients

Healthy food doesn't have to be complicated. In fact, it often isn't. This circles back to the previous conversation about searching for food with short ingredient lists. Whole foods are simply themselves. An apple is an apple. A decent nut butter includes only ground nuts and maybe sea salt. Straightforward, honest food leaves nothing for producers and manufacturers to hide behind. By focusing on simple, quality ingredients, you can't really go wrong. You don't have to do anything to a ripe peach to make it taste good in late summer at the peak of its season. But when considering something like artificial cheese spread, a highly processed, man-made food, more ingredients and complex processes are needed to create something people will accept and like.

7. Seasonal Foods

Due to the globalization of our food supply, we have access to almost any food at any time of the year. In so many ways, this is the ultimate convenience. Unfortunately, it also draws us away from the natural rhythm of our local climate and many other benefits.

Nutritionally, studies have found that plants specifically, such as broccoli, that are grown and harvested in season actually produce more antioxidants and anti-inflammatory properties than those grown out of season. Although this is not the case for every edible plant, it does apply to many.

Seasonal foods may also support our seasonal health needs. It's a concept that intuitively makes sense to me, although more research is needed on this subject. For example, vitamin C–rich citrus is in season during the peak of cold and flu season in the winter months, whereas leafy greens are seasonally

How Can I Tell What Produce Is in Season?

One way to help you identify what produce is in season is to consider the life cycle of a plant. First, ask yourself if your fruit or vegetable is a root (such as a carrot), a flower (broccoli), or a fruit (tomato). Start at the ground level or the roots of a plant and work your way up to the flower or fruit. You can't grow a flower without growing its roots first, right? Roots like onions, potatoes, and beets stay insulated in the cold weather tucked away in the ground, but can you imagine baby broccoli sprouts trying to survive the winter? It is highly unlikely that they could. As the weather improves and the soil begins to warm in the early spring, shoots, baby greens, and herbs start to grow. Next, in late spring, the first full-grown greens and delicate fruits like strawberries arrive. Can you see we're climbing up the plant as the weather warms? As days get longer and the summer sun shines brighter, out pop the tomatoes, cucumbers, peaches, and plums—fruit that grows higher on the plant and requires the roots, stalks, and flowers to produce.

abundant and available in the spring and summer months when our bodies benefit most from natural detoxification.

Foods grown and harvested in season typically have better flavor and texture as well as more vibrant color. Their growth needs fewer interventions and resources, like water and fertilizer or electricity for heat lamps, that use up more of our precious natural resources. Harvesting and consuming foods in season can also minimize our exposure to toxic chemicals and pesticides that are more readily used with foods grown and harvested out of season.

Finally, food that is grown and harvested in season tends to be less expensive. When supply is up, prices are down, a concept known as supply and demand. Remembering this will help you save money, especially when buying organic foods. We can also support our local economy and community when we choose to buy seasonal foods, since they are in abundance and typically travel shorter distances.

Learning what food is in season and when can be a daunting task, though. A great place to start is at your local farmer's market. Walking around, you will inevitably start to notice what's in season without having to look too far. The farmers bring their current crops and bounty to the market, often displaying what they have harvested that week or even that day. (Please refer to Appendix A for a seasonal produce chart.)

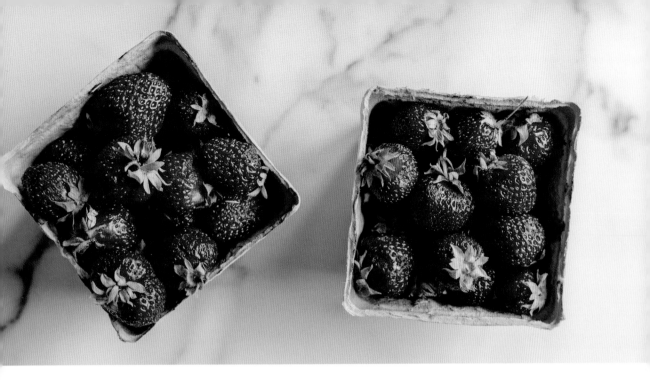

Small farmers who sell seasonal foods at farmer's markets are 10 percent more likely to stay in business compared to those who don't. Buying from small farmers supports your local community while also promoting a better food system.

8. Bonus! Foods That Give Back

Wouldn't it be amazing if everything we purchased and ate somehow gave back to people and the planet in some way? Although this is nearly impossible at the moment, many food and brand choices we make can do just that. It's not enough anymore to just buy your favorite brand. You have a responsibility to support your local and global community, especially if you're eating and using their resources. We have to stop thinking someone else will care. It's our duty to think beyond ourselves and support organizations that are making an impact and working for change. Even if you choose to buy only *one* food brand that gives back, you're making a difference.

As previously described, buying organic produce is one way you can help reduce environmental pollution and greenhouse gas emissions. But

FAIR TRADE CERTIFIED

what else can you do to make an impact? Look for products that help establish school gardens, support wildlife conservation, or sustain tropical forests. Buying Fair Trade Certified products, for example, is an excellent way to support sustainability, community, and environmental stewardship. Look for the Fair Trade Certified label on international imports and foods like chocolate, coffee, coconut oil, and more. Put this into practice and use Fair Trade Certified chocolate in the Flourless Chocolate Almond Butter Brownies (page 161) or the Chocolate Tofu Mousse with Coconut Whip (page 182).

It's Not Just What You Eat

So far, it's been all about the food, but *what* we eat is only one part of the story. *How* we eat is the other. How we eat is an integral part of finding balance and transforming our food into medicine. You can do everything in your power to get quality food to your plate, but if you don't consider how you're eating that food, then what's the point? Literally, how we eat our food is how it turns into our medicine. So if you're going to dedicate precious time and energy to finding quality foods, I encourage you to also find the time and energy to consider quality ways in which to enjoy that food.

Slow Down

These two words may be the best recommendation I offer in this entire book. We're obsessed with getting things done. We're constantly on the move and are flying around, attempting to check off another box and cross off another to-do item before another day is over. We are celebrated when we get more done, and we wear "busy" like a badge of honor. We eat in a hurry or on the go, and we skip meals. We rarely slow down until we come to a crashing stop when our bodies are severely stressed, and we get sick or are forced to slow down for another—usually negative—reason. I'm guilty of this too. My husband says I have octopus arms that can juggle eight things at once, but does that mean I should use them all day every day?

Anxiety, shallow breathing, increased heart rate, restlessness, decreased digestion, poor-quality sleep, irritability—these are all symptoms of fight-or-flight, of the sympathetic nervous system taking over. This is a stress response that our bodies actually use intentionally to protect us from imminent danger, like running from a bear, for example. In this state, the sympathetic nervous system is preparing the body for physical and mental activity to keep us out of

> ### The Twenty-Minute Challenge
>
> An activity I give to most of my patients, but particularly those with digestive issues, is what I call the Twenty-Minute Challenge. Try this at your next meal. Your challenge is to take twenty minutes or more to eat your meal. You can't rush through and save the last bite for the end. You have to portion out your food and eat it slowly throughout the twenty minutes. You can't watch TV or look at your phone during this time. No reading or writing. Just be. Be present with your food—and your company, if you're sharing your meal with someone. Take note of how you feel before and after. How does this experience differ from your typical mealtime? Does your food taste any different? Are you hungry or full afterward? Do you feel more grounded? This is an excellent tool to help you slow down.

harm's way. It's ingenious, really. Our hearts beat faster and stronger to pump more blood to our extremities, additional blood glucose becomes available for our muscles and tissues, our airways open wider, our pupils dilate, and our blood pressure increases, all in an effort to help us run away from that bear. The problem is, though, we're just running our errands.

Many of us live under constant stress. We may spend months and years in this state, which eventually takes its toll in the form of digestive distress, high blood pressure, metabolic and hormonal imbalances, and even chronic disease. I mention this because the first thing we must change about how we eat is to slow down. We have to make room for balance and carve out time to care for ourselves. This can mean different things for different people, but I'm certain it's where we all must begin. This is a similar concept to the first principle of food as medicine, as stated previously. We must make a conscious decision and commitment to care for ourselves, then the rest can follow.

The opposite of the sympathetic nervous system is the parasympathetic nervous system, which is responsible for our bodily functions when we are in a state of rest. This is also called rest-and-digest mode, as it activates different metabolic processes, decreases our heart rate, relaxes our muscles, and stimulates digestion. It is an ideal state to be in when eating. If you're relaxed when you eat, you will adequately chew your food, allowing you to digest it better, feel hunger and fullness more readily, and assimilate more nutrients—all important factors for optimal nutrition and health. You may even alleviate gastric pain and other gastrointestinal (GI) issues caused by poor digestion.

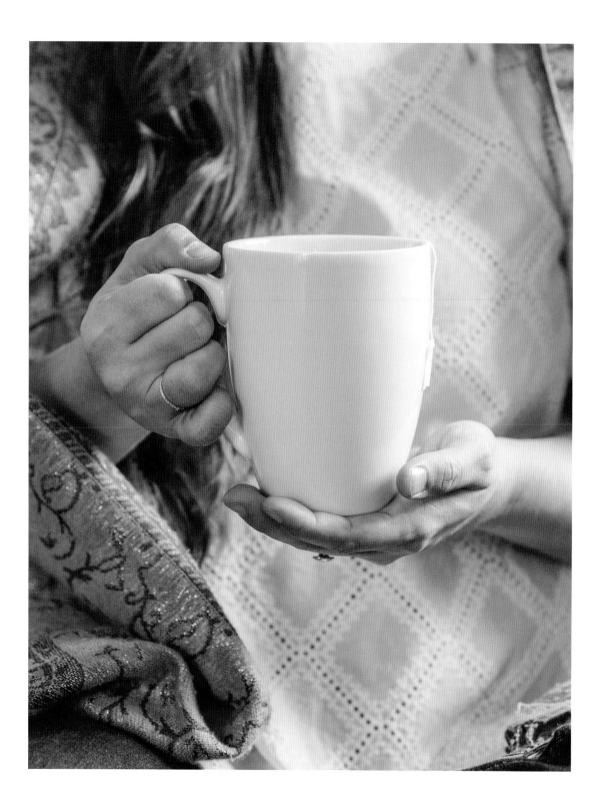

Offering yourself more time to eat your next meal is a great place to start. Maybe you can commit to actually eating breakfast for two days next week before running out the door or to making a nice meal at home tonight instead of grabbing take-out again. These are all realistic places to start and incredible ways to slow down, reconnect with yourself and others, and become more present. The positive impact this one fairly simple activity can have on your health is remarkable, and the ripple effect is undeniably contagious.

Be Mindful

The concept of mindfulness continues to gain popularity and for good reason. As technology takes over and our lives speed up, we are desperately in need of an antidote for the anxiety, stress, insomnia, and other negative health conditions we face at an ever-growing rate. Mindfulness is a fantastic tool to help us combat the stressors of life and can be individualized and accessed at all hours of the day, everywhere we go.

By definition, mindfulness is a state of open and active attention on the present moment. Without judgment, you observe your thoughts and feelings *right now*. Mindfulness anchors you in the present and awakens you to your current experience. Some people practice this in the form of seated meditation or deep breathing exercises. I like to practice mindfulness in my kitchen while cooking and at my dining room table before and during my meals.

When we bring mindfulness to our kitchens, plates, and thus ourselves while eating, we call this "mindful eating." This is one of the most effective ways to nourish yourself and turn your food into medicine. Mindful eating includes cooking and eating without distractions, slowing down, noting and engaging your senses, coping with emotional eating, listening to your hunger and fullness cues, and observing how food affects your mood and body. These actions have been researched as means to improve digestion, decrease anxiety related to eating, minimize binge eating and other eating disorder behaviors, improve overall mood, support healthy weight loss, and more.

Diligently kneading bread with your hands, thoroughly investigating a colorful piece of fruit, or lovingly admiring the flavors of your favorite food all require mindfulness. These activities call on us to live in the present. They encourage us to leave fight-or-flight mode and bring us back into our bodies, grounding us in the current moment. What a beautiful thing!

A recent report from the USDA found that the average American spends two-and-a-half hours eating every day while spending half of that time also driving, watching TV, or doing another involved and distracting activity. Now let's be realistic; some days this is all we can manage. I challenge you, though, to consider when this is *really* necessary and when you can practice mindful eating and mindful meal preparation instead. Can you identify when in your day you could benefit most from mindful eating?

When you're ready to practice mindful eating, here are some helpful tips:

- **Create a space that you use only for food preparation and/or eating.** Designating a specific place, like your kitchen table, will help you register that as the place you go when it's time to eat. Try not to use your kitchen counter as a mail collector or work on your laptop at your dining room table. The thought is, if you separate your spaces, over time you can minimize the distractions that occur there and will instead be triggered to prepare meals or eat—and nothing else—when in those spaces. You're also setting healthy boundaries, which will allow for greater success in the future.

- **Take a deep breath.** Before you start cooking or eating, take six deep breaths. By doing this, research shows that you're physiologically activating your parasympathetic nervous system, which is responsible for helping you to rest and digest. How cool is that? It's like your own personal, built-in reboot button.

- **Sit down when eating.** Pause and take a break from life to enjoy your meal fully. Sitting down can help you transition into a more intentional and restful place, aiding in that transition to rest-and-digest mode.

- **Turn off all technology.** Remove any unnecessary distractions and become present, so you can focus your whole being on what's in front of you—your food.

- **Offer thanks for your food.** Thank all the people, animals, plants, and resources that came together to create your nourishing meal. By pausing and reflecting on this before enjoying your food, you are bringing intention and awareness to it. You are becoming more mindful.

- **Use all of your senses.** Spend five minutes observing your food using all five of your senses—sight, smell, sound, taste, and touch. Give each sensory experience one minute of your time. How does the food look up close? Notice anything new? How does it smell? Can you describe the texture or flavor? Does it make a sound? You get the idea. You may be surprised at what you observe and how you feel after this exercise.

- **Chew your food well.** Most of us inhale our food in mere minutes, often not chewing it adequately first. This leads to indigestion or slow digestion and gastrointestinal discomfort, and it deprives the brain of time to catch up and assess our true hunger and fullness level. Now you don't have to chew each bite thirty-plus times until it's completely puréed, but bring your awareness to chewing and see how that changes your experience with your food and digestion.

- **Allow yourself time.** Stay seated for a few minutes after finishing your meal. Converse with your company or reflect to yourself about how satisfactory your meal was. Take a deep breath and take your time before jumping up from the table and getting back to your fast-paced life.

Practice Mindful Eating When Eating Out

This is not hard to do actually, and it has been shown to significantly increase food and diet-related self-efficacy. Here are some tips I give to my patients when eating out:

- Show up at the restaurant with moderate, not intense, hunger.

- Review the menu online beforehand to minimize social distractions or peer pressure when you're at the restaurant.

- Choose a balanced meal that includes healthy fats, protein, and carbohydrates.

- Add a salad or side dish to your order, if necessary, to create more balance.

- Take subtle, deep breaths to check in and ground yourself before eating.

- Put down your utensil between each bite or often throughout the meal.

- Chew slowly and savor your food.

- Check in with yourself partway through your meal and assess your hunger/fullness level on a scale from 1 to 10.

- When you're full, stop eating and take any leftovers home to enjoy at another time.

Find Joy

Of course, food is a source of nourishment, but it is also a source of joy. Certain nutrients, like vitamin B12, provide the building blocks for neurotransmitters that contribute to good mood and happiness and can even decrease depression. But outside of nutrition, there are many other ways that food can inspire joy.

Sharing food with loved ones, friends, new acquaintances, and everyone in between offers us an opportunity to connect and relate to others regardless of our differences. Parents can find contentment knowing they've provided their child with adequate food and nutrition. Eating can offer a sense of safety for some or evoke happy memories for others. Cooking and feeding people can be stimulating and exciting. Food can even elicit a sexual connection with another person or be visually pleasing and, thus, a source of artful inspiration for both the chef and the diner.

Whatever it may be, I encourage you to find your source of joy in the kitchen or on your plate, because food can't only be about science and nourishing our bodies. Research shows that when joy is removed from our eating experiences, disordered eating, indigestion, and inadequate nutrient intake are just a few of the negative outcomes.

Honor Your Feelings without Food

This is really challenging. Food is inherently emotional. Food is love. Food is celebratory. Food is security. And these are not "bad" things! Remember, emotional eating is a normal human experience. Many of us eat out of boredom, anxiety, stress, depression—the list goes on. But what happens when we use food as our *only* means for coping with our emotions? Overeating or binge eating, digestive distress, and high blood pressure are just a few concerns raised by using food as the only coping mechanism.

If this is something you can relate to, I encourage you to ask yourself a few basic questions:

- Are you head hungry or body hungry? This question is really asking you where your hunger comes from. Has it been a while since you ate something (body hunger), or did you just receive some stressful news (head hunger)?

- If you're not body (physiologically) hungry, what's your dominant emotion? What are you really feeling?

- Once you identify your true emotion(s), what would help you cope with that emotion that does not include food or eating? Do you need sleep? Do you need a break from work?

- Have your basic needs been met? Do you need more rest? Do you feel heard in your relationship(s)? Are you receiving respect and love from others? These are all important needs that must be met in order for us to heal from emotional eating cycles.

- If emotional eating is something you struggle with, consider finding outside support. There are many qualified professionals who can help you work through this. I recommend seeking counseling from a registered dietitian nutritionist who supports Intuitive Eating and/ or disordered eating therapies or from a licensed mental health counselor who specializes in emotional eating.

2

FINDING
BALANCE

Know when to push. Know when to pause.

DR. AVIVA ROMM, PHYSICIAN, MIDWIFE, AND HERBALIST

GOOD HEALTH is a condition of being sound in the body, mind, and spirit. Your effort is minimal, and the outcome is maximal. You're at ease and free from pain. You have energy, find pleasure easily, are inspired creatively, and are stimulated intellectually. You've found balance. You've found your equilibrium.

When I think of living in balance, I picture one of those stacking rock sculptures. Just as we are unique beings, each sculpture is a combination of unique stones placed together with intention and forethought to create a work of art—a balanced structure. No two sculptures are alike, although they all require similar qualities—such as awareness, concentration, and dedication—to make. We, too, have individualized needs, yet we may also benefit from similar recommendations.

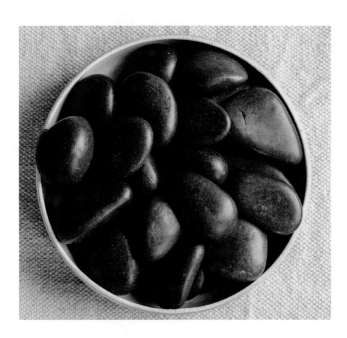

Over time, and at various life stages, the conditions for balance and your personal equilibrium will change. Physiologically, your nutrient needs, organ function, and physical ability will change. Your emotional intelligence, motivation, and overall mental health will evolve. You may even cultivate a new spiritual awareness or understanding as you age. So many factors will change; thus, your overall state of health and balance will too.

We can all agree, though, that good nutrition is a key component to health throughout all of life's stages. Again, the specifics, such as diet composition and the necessary amount of certain nutrients and sources, will be different for everyone, but some basic rules will apply (see Appendix B for Dietary Reference Intakes). We all need macronutrients and micronutrients to survive and thrive, for example.

In this chapter, I've highlighted some elementary yet significant nutritional information, including valuable details on vitamins and minerals, essential food groups, and inspiration for creating a balanced plate whether you're an omnivore, vegetarian, or vegan.

Macronutrients

Macronutrients make up the bulk of our diet and supply us with energy and essential nutrients. There are three main macronutrients we must consume for optimal health: proteins, fats, and carbohydrates. Each group yields a different amount of energy per gram consumed (proteins = 4 calories/gram, fats = 9 calories/gram, carbohydrates = 4 calories/gram), and each is composed of various subgroups.

Proteins

Proteins are responsible for most of the structural components of our cells. They're needed for tissue maintenance and replacement, function, and growth. They also help to create enzymes, membranes, transporters, and some hormones.

When we eat protein from animals or plants, it's broken down into amino acids and peptides, which become the building blocks of the various functions and structures in the body. Of the twenty amino acids used to make proteins, nine are essential and must be provided by our diet compared to the others that are nonessential and that our bodies can make on their own.

Complete proteins are proteins, typically from animal sources, that naturally contain all nine essential amino acids. Incomplete proteins, typically from plant sources, are missing essential amino acids and must be combined with another incomplete protein that has a different arrangement of amino acids to create a complete profile or "complementary protein."

Fats

Fats are involved with neurological development and growth, tissue repair, absorption of fat-soluble vitamins and vitamin precursors, and hormone production. One of the main roles of fats, though, is to serve as an energy source for the body, given that fat contains 9 calories per gram compared to the 4 calories per gram of proteins and carbohydrates.

There are three types of fat: unsaturated fats, which include monounsaturated and polyunsaturated; saturated fats; and trans fats. Monounsaturated and polyunsaturated fats are found mostly in plants and are liquid at room temperature. Saturated fats are most common in animal fats, but can also be found in some plants, and are solid at room temperature. Trans fats are mostly manufactured from hydrogenated vegetable oils and found in highly processed foods, although they can also be found naturally at very low levels in some animal fats. Interestingly enough, the FDA recently banned the production of man-made trans fat due to the direct and dangerous correlation between trans fats and heart disease, high cholesterol, and obesity.

The body requires "healthy fats" (monounsaturated and polyunsaturated) for optimal function. Monounsaturated fats are heart-healthy fats that help to reduce cholesterol, benefit insulin levels, and help to regulate blood sugar. Polyunsaturated fats are best known for their essential fatty acid composition (omega-3 and omega-6 fatty acids), which we must obtain from food as our bodies do not synthesize these fats. Specifically, omega-3 fatty acids are composed of alpha-linolenic acid (ALA), docosahexaenoic acid (DHA), and eicosapentaenoic acid (EPA), which are incredibly beneficial for mental health; cardiovascular health; prevention of autoimmune disease, cancer, and inflammation; bone and joint health; sleep quality; infant and child growth and development; eye health; skin health; and overall aging.

Carbohydrates

Carbohydrates are a major source of energy, especially for the brain and central nervous system. They also help to preserve muscle mass, promote healthy digestion and heart health, and manage blood glucose levels.

Carbohydrates are found naturally in plant-based foods and dairy and are broken down into polysaccharides, oligosaccharides, disaccharides, and monosaccharides, also known as glucose. Some carbohydrates also contain non-digestible dietary fiber that helps to lower cholesterol, manage blood glucose levels, and promote digestive health and regular elimination. There is also functional fiber or isolated and extracted fiber that's manufactured and added to foods to help boost consumer intake.

Micronutrients

Micronutrients are vitamins and minerals or chemical compounds found in the foods we eat. We must consume micronutrients directly from plants, which obtain nutrients from the soil, or animal sources since our bodies only make some vitamins and do not naturally make minerals. Depending on where we live, we can find some micronutrients in our drinking water, also known as mineral water. Micronutrients are essential to our health as they keep us energized, support growth and development, produce enzymes and hormones, aid in digestion and metabolism, strengthen bones, help repair tissues, preserve and improve mental health, prevent deficiencies and diseases, slow oxidative damage, and so much more.

Vitamins, specifically, are categorized as either fat-soluble (dissolves in fat) or water-soluble (dissolves in water). Fat-soluble vitamins are stored in the liver and fat tissue and are eliminated more slowly than water-soluble vitamins, which are not stored by the body. Fat-soluble vitamins include vitamins A, D, E, and K, while all others are water-soluble. For optimal absorption, it's best to eat fat-soluble, vitamin-rich foods with a healthy source of fat, such as nuts, seeds, coconut oil, and so on. Water-soluble vitamins are easily absorbed with most foods.

Vitamins

Your body is a complex and well-functioning machine, although it needs some help acquiring all necessary vitamins from food and/or supplements (aka essential vitamins). It's important that we have the required vitamins onboard so that our bodies can perform optimally. Below is a list of essential vitamins A through K describing their functions and actions in the body.

- VITAMIN A is a vitamin and antioxidant. It is an essential nutrient for vision, immunity, growth and development, skin health, female and male reproductive function, and red blood cell production. It also helps your body fight free radical damage, reduce inflammation, and prevent premature aging.

- VITAMIN B1 (THIAMIN) is necessary for energy production, metabolism, and nerve function.

- VITAMIN B2 (RIBOFLAVIN) is essential for a healthy pregnancy, energy production, detoxification, and the metabolism of other vitamins and minerals. Specifically, we need an adequate intake of riboflavin to produce the enzymes needed to process vitamin B6 and folate.

- VITAMIN B3 (NIACIN) is needed for energy production and metabolism, as well as DNA repair and antioxidant protection.

- VITAMIN B5 (PANTOTHENIC ACID) is involved in overall energy metabolism and fat metabolism.

- VITAMIN B6 (PYRIDOXINE) is necessary for the production of red blood cells, carbohydrate metabolism, hormone function, brain and nervous system health, and liver detoxification. Vitamin B6 consumption and/or supplementation has also been associated with improved heart health and decreased nausea during pregnancy.

- VITAMIN B7 (BIOTIN) helps to balance blood sugar, improve skin health, regulate gene expression, and may even prevent neurological degeneration.

- VITAMIN B9 (FOLATE) promotes brain and nervous system health and development, DNA metabolism, protein metabolism, cardiovascular health, red blood cell production, reproductive health (decreased neural tube defects), and may even decrease the risk of cancer, especially breast and colorectal cancer. Folate depends on vitamin B$_{12}$ to be absorbed, stored, and metabolized, so consider adding B$_{12}$-rich foods to your meals and snacks while consuming sources of folate. Folic acid is the synthetic form of folate found in fortified foods and vitamin supplements.

- VITAMIN B$_{12}$ (COBALAMIN) promotes cardiovascular health, brain and nervous system health, and DNA production, and it is required for folate metabolism. Vitamin B$_{12}$ consumption and supplementation also treats pernicious anemia and may prevent some forms of cancer.

- VITAMIN C (ASCORBIC ACID) functions as a powerful antioxidant, plays a vital role in collagen production, enhances immune function, reduces blood pressure, promotes cardiovascular health, promotes brain health, and may reduce the risk for cataracts and certain types of cancer.

- VITAMIN D is a vitamin that functions as a hormone. It helps to regulate blood sugar, boost immune function, promote healthy bone development and density, decrease inflammation, promote fetal health, absorb calcium and phosphorus, regulate blood pressure, decrease the risk of cancer, and prevent cognitive decline.

- VITAMIN E functions as an antioxidant and protects against heart disease, cancer, cataracts, and macular degeneration. It may also help to prevent cognitive impairment, improve immune function, and enhance insulin response.

- VITAMIN K plays an important role in blood clotting, supports beneficial bone metabolism, increases cardiovascular health, improves vascular health, and encourages various other cellular functions.

Minerals

Similarly to vitamins, our bodies need minerals to perform different functions. There are two sub-types: macrominerals (calcium, magnesium, phosphorus, potassium, sodium) and trace minerals (chromium, copper, fluoride, iodine, iron, manganese, molybdenum, selenium, zinc). Below is a list of both types of minerals found in food.

- CALCIUM is an important mineral and electrolyte that supports bone and dental health, regulates pH balance in the body, and helps control muscle and nerve function. Calcium can also reduce the risk for preeclampsia in pregnant women and may lower the risk of developing colorectal cancer. Vitamin D is required for optimal calcium absorption, so consider adding a vitamin D–containing food source when eating calcium-rich foods.

- CHROMIUM plays a key role in normal insulin function and blood sugar control.

- COPPER is involved in energy production, iron metabolism, immune system function, connective tissue development, and brain and nervous system function.

- FLUORIDE is an important structural component of teeth and bones. It can help to reverse early signs of tooth decay and prevent the growth of oral bacteria.

- IODINE is a main component for thyroid health and hormones that support normal growth, metabolism, and neurological development. It's also an important mineral for regulating body temperature and supporting healthy reproductive function in both women and men.

- IRON is an essential nutrient that supports many biological functions, such as energy production, DNA synthesis, red blood cell production, and oxygen transport in the blood. Iron also supports normal immune function and antioxidant enzymes. There are two forms of iron: heme and non-heme. Heme iron is found in animal foods, and non-heme iron is primarily found in plant foods. Heme iron is more readily absorbed by the body compared to non-heme iron. Consuming vitamin C with any iron-rich foods, but especially plant sources or non-heme iron, can help to optimize iron absorption.

- MAGNESIUM is an electrolyte and cofactor for more than three hundred enzymes and is involved with many important biological functions, such as food metabolism, synthesis of fats and proteins, DNA synthesis, intracellular communication, muscle function, bone density, and learning and memory function.

- MANGANESE facilitates bone development and wound healing; helps with protein, carbohydrate, and cholesterol metabolism; and is a key player in antioxidant function.

- MOLYBDENUM functions to metabolize protein, DNA, and other foreign compounds. It also maintains sulfur balance in the body and helps with antioxidant function.

- PHOSPHORUS makes up a structural component of bones and teeth, cell membranes, and DNA. It also assists in energy production and fluid and pH balance.

- POTASSIUM is an essential mineral and electrolyte that helps maintain fluid balance in the body. It's required for optimal nerve function and muscle contractions and influences blood pressure and blood volume.

- SELENIUM is needed for thyroid hormone production, assists in normal antioxidant function, and supports a healthy immune system.

Food or Supplement?

This is a question I often hear from my patients. Ideally, you can meet your nutritional needs from a well-balanced diet rather than supplements, although supplementation may be necessary for some, and has been shown to be therapeutic for prevention and treatment of some acute and chronic diseases. Supplements are highly recommended for pregnant women, vegans and some vegetarians, elderly people, people with medical conditions, or nutrient deficiencies, and anyone who has a restrictive diet for any reason.

Eating vitamins and minerals in a whole foods diet has its benefits, including a more diverse and robust nutrient profile, the addition of natural fiber from the food, and more antioxidants and other phytonutrients compared to singular supplements. There's also something called food synergy, which is the concept that vitamins and minerals, as well as other food constituents, are absorbed and perform better when delivered in combination with other nutrients in food rather than isolated as a single nutrient in supplement form. Research actually shows this to be true: isolated nutrients are generally less effective and sometimes even harmful compared to their food-based counterparts.

- SODIUM is an electrolyte that helps to control blood pressure and volume, as well as fluid volume outside cells. Sodium and chloride work together to regulate blood pressure and control extracellular volume.

- ZINC is an essential mineral for many physiological functions. It regulates gene expression and cell signaling, influences hormones, assists in hemoglobin production and the oxygen-carrying capacity of red blood cells, and supports a healthy immune system.

For a list of vitamin and mineral food sources, please refer to the nutrient index in Appendix C.

Rainbow Food

Eating "rainbow food" refers to eating a colorful diet. For many of us, it may be easier and even more pleasing to eat monochromatic foods, especially tan, white, and brown foods, such as bread, rice, cheese, crackers, and other convenient foods that taste good but have less nutrients. As we learn more about food, we are finding that naturally colorful foods may actually deliver more health benefits, specifically more phytonutrients such as antioxidants and other health-promoting constituents. Many of these nutrients have disease-preventing and even cancer-fighting properties. By maintaining a varied and colorful whole foods diet, you are laying the foundation for nutritional success. Can you get a minimum of three colors on the plate at your next meal? Try making the Rainbow Rolls with Ginger Almond Sauce (page 153) or Vegetable Fried Brown Rice with Ginger Sauce (page 133) for a rainbow color explosion!

RED FOODS such as tomatoes, pink grapefruit, watermelon, and guava are often rich in vitamin C and lycopene, which are both powerful antioxidants. Red foods also contain polyphenols, which help to reduce inflammation and maintain a healthy gut barrier.

ORANGE/YELLOW FOODS such as carrots, squash, cantaloupe, and mango are rich in beta-carotene and vitamin C, which act as antioxidants, support healthy vision, and promote a healthy immune system. Orange/yellow foods may also help to prevent some forms of cancer.

YELLOW/GREEN FOODS such as kiwis, avocados, and pistachios typically contain lutein, which is beneficial for eye health, and vitamin C, which is most notable for its antioxidant and immune system support.

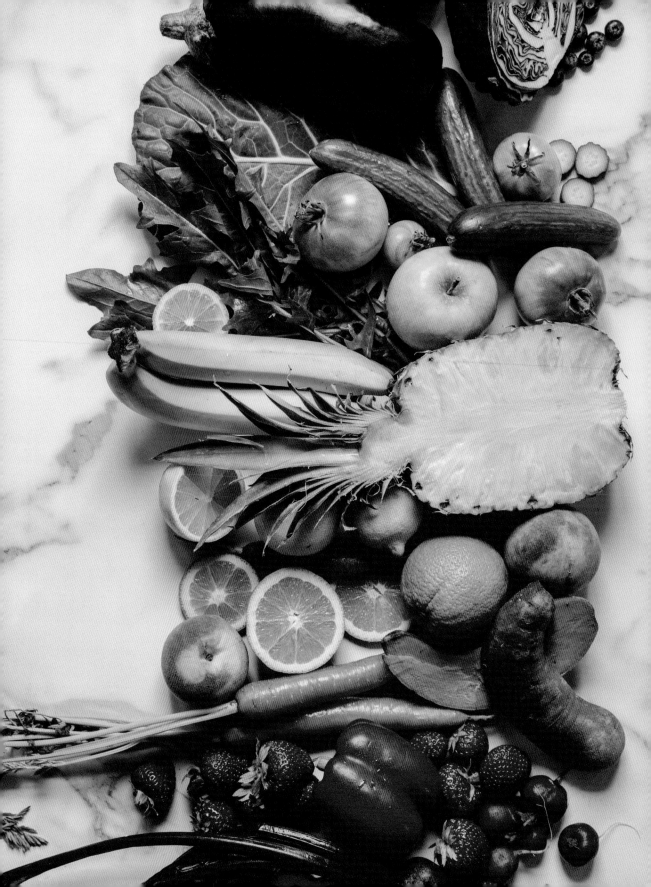

GREEN FOODS such as kale, broccoli, brussel sprouts, and bok choy are naturally rich in chlorophyll and isothiocyanates, which help the body to detox naturally. They're also rich in vitamin K, folate, potassium, omega-3 fatty acids, and carotenoids, which perform a variety of biological functions, including forming blood clots, preventing neural tube defects during fetal development, lowering blood pressure, and even protecting against some forms of cancer.

BLUE/PURPLE foods such as eggplant, blueberries, plums, pomegranates, and blackberries contain anthocyanins, which are beneficial for heart health and maintaining healthy blood pressure. The darker the blue or purple (and oftentimes deep red), the richer the anthocyanin concentration.

Essential Food Groups

There are a lot of opinions out there about which food groups are and are not essential for good health. In your lifetime, thus far, you've likely heard many different diet recommendations. Theories of some of the more popular fad diets, which are not founded on research, include "only eat raw fruits and veg-etables," "avoid carbohydrates entirely," and "ketosis is the optimal state for our bodies at all times." You've likely seen various food pyramids and graphs explaining the perfect diet. It's a challenge to wade through the murky waters of diet culture and flashy food trends to find what really works best for you. But that's precisely it—the core of my recommendation here is to find what works for *you*! After all, you know your body best.

I've summarized important details of common food groups—and some uncommon ones too—that I think are worthy of discussion. Again, this infor-mation is a guide, not a rule. Take what works, leave the rest.

Fruits and Vegetables
Technically speaking, fruits are edible, seed-bearing foods from flowering plants, and vegetables are all other parts of an edible plant, including the roots, stems, and leaves. In a culinary context, and in most grocery stores and home kitchens, savory fruits such as tomatoes, eggplants, and zucchini are considered vegetables.

Eating fruits and vegetables can reduce your risk for some chronic dis-eases. They contain essential nutrients, including dietary fiber and important vitamins like potassium and vitamin C. A diet rich in fruits and vegetables is shown to reduce your risk for heart disease, heart attack, and stroke, while

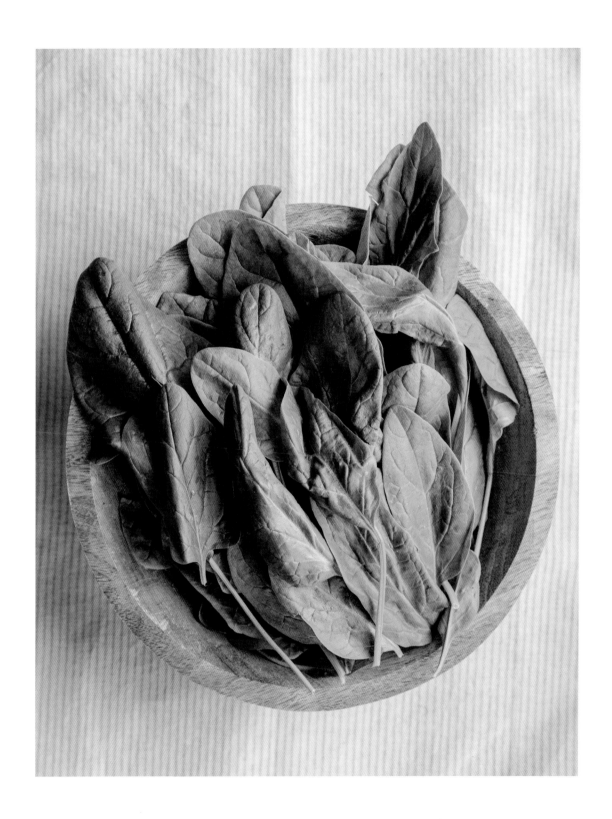

also protecting you against some forms of cancer, obesity, type 2 diabetes, high blood pressure, kidney stones, and bone loss.

Leafy greens almost deserve their own category or food group. They are technically part of the vegetable category, but they pack an additional nutritious punch. Lutein, vitamin K, calcium, fiber, magnesium, folate, and iron are just some of the extra nutrients they contain. Leafy greens, especially bitter ones like arugula, dandelion, and kale, for example, also activate taste buds and stimulate enzyme production and bile flow for healthy digestion while promoting natural detoxification.

Grains

Grains are individual hard, dry seeds that are harvested from a variety of grain crops or plants and are consumed in whole (fresh and dried) and refined or processed forms. Whole grains contain all of the original edible parts of the grain, also called the grain kernel, like wild rice or barley. Refined grains such as white rice or all-purpose flour have been processed to remove the bran and germ, give the grain a refined and softer texture, and improve the shelf life.

Whole grains are loaded with many important nutrients, including fiber, B vitamins, and minerals such as iron and magnesium. Consider at least half of your grain intake to be whole grains rather than refined ones for increased health. Whole grains have been shown to reduce blood cholesterol levels, heart disease, obesity, and type 2 diabetes. Fiber from grains also maintains healthy bowel function, reduces constipation, and helps provide a feeling of fullness from fewer calories.

Protein

Protein comes from both animal and plant sources. Meat, poultry, seafood, eggs, dairy, beans/legumes, soy, nuts, and seeds are all considered sources of protein. Animal-derived proteins typically have more available protein bite for bite, although there are substantial amounts of protein in plant foods, such as soybeans, as well. Although there are small amounts of protein in vegetables, the amount is minimal and should not be considered your only source of protein.

Both animal and plant proteins contain other nutrients such as B vitamins, iron, zinc, and vitamin E, which function as building blocks for enzymes, hormones, vitamins, bones, muscles, cartilage, skin, and blood. And plant proteins specifically may reduce the risk of heart disease.

Is It OK to Eat Soy?

As a registered dietitian nutritionist, this is another common question I am often asked. Soy is a highly disputed food. Many people believe it causes cancer, especially breast cancer, due to its phytoestrogen content. As a big fan of soy, I'm always so pleased to debunk myths about this remarkable food!

- **There is no association between eating soy and breast cancer.** In a recent study looking at nine thousand breast cancer survivors, eating soy actually lowered the risk of breast cancer recurrence, even in women with estrogen-receptor-positive tumors. The American Cancer Society states that a moderate consumption of soy foods is safe and may even be beneficial.

- **Soy does not lower testosterone in men.** Most concerns related to soy's "emasculating effects" come from studies conducted on rats and mice, not humans. Rodents metabolize soy differently than humans, making this comparison inapplicable.

- **Eating soy foods does not cause hypothyroidism.** Only one study found that women who were taking high phytoestrogen soy supplements and already had subclinical hypothyroidism had issues with soy and hypothyroidism. When soy is consumed at a moderate level in the diet as opposed to in high and concentrated amounts in supplements, there is no evidence that it causes hypothyroidism.

Recent and quality research shows that soy may actually have anticancer and heart-healthy properties, prevent hypertension and diabetes, as well as help to relieve negative symptoms during menopause.

In general, I highly recommend organic whole soy foods (tempeh, tofu, edamame, soy milk). Remember though, these are different from soy products (soy isolates, soy isoflavones), which I recommend you minimize or eliminate completely. Whole soy foods are a great source of plant protein—one of the highest. They also contain fiber, calcium, and omega-3 fatty acids (healthy fats). My preferred form of soy is fermented, specifically tempeh. Not only does the fermentation process help with digestion, but it also reduces the phytic acid content that can prevent mineral malabsorption. Check out the recipe for The Simplest Tempeh Tacos with Whole Wheat and Flax Tortillas (page 155). Other beloved fermented soy foods include miso, shoyu, tamari, and natto.

Fats and Oils

Fats and oils aren't necessarily their own food group, but they do provide essential nutrients such as monounsaturated and polyunsaturated fatty acids (healthy fats), so in my opinion they deserve their own category. They are processed from both plant and animal sources such as olives and salmon.

Fats provide a major source of energy and help us to absorb fat-soluble vitamins. Fats support and build cell membranes and the insulating layer that surrounds the nerves. However, omega-3 fatty acids are the real star in the healthy fat category. They have been shown to help build cell membranes and influence cell receptors; produce hormones; support infant health and development; prevent and even treat heart disease and stroke; reduce blood pressure; raise high-density lipoprotein (HDL), or "good cholesterol"; lower triglycerides; improve cognitive function; decrease the risk of vision loss in older adults; reduce inflammation, especially in people with rheumatoid arthritis; and possibly even lower the risk of some forms of cancer. *Powerful stuff.*

Fermented and Cultured Foods

Fermentation is a metabolic process that occurs in the absence of oxygen to create acids, gases, and alcohol. Organisms or bacteria spontaneously establish themselves on or in foods and initiate fermentation, creating tangy probiotic-rich foods such as sauerkraut and kimchi.

Cultured foods require a "culture" or bacterial "starter" to begin the process of fermentation, such as with commercial yogurt and some cheese. Cultured foods are also considered fermented foods. Vegetables, fruits, grains, milk, meats, seafood, and beans can all be fermented. Check out the recipe for Cultured Key Lime Cashew Yogurt (page 143) for a great example of a cultured food.

Fermentation predigests food into more elemental or basic forms, allowing for more easily digestible components. For example, fermented meat and fish are tenderized and lactose in milk converts to lactic acid, increasing digestibility (that's why some lactose-intolerant people can digest yogurt without any issues). Fermented foods also increase levels of B vitamins and may even help to convert foods into anticancer compounds such as isothiocyanates. Fermentation can also transform some foods into less toxic versions of themselves; for example, by increasing the solubility of phytates found in grains, legumes, seeds, and nuts or by reducing pesticide residue on vegetables.

Finally, fermented foods contribute live bacterial cultures or probiotics— aka healthy bacteria—to our microbiomes, which are a collection of more than one thousand species of microbes that live in the body, particularly in the large intestine. They positively contribute to many of our necessary metabolic functions, protect us from harmful pathogens, help us digest our food, produce crucial vitamins, defend our immune systems, and positively affect many other physiological functions. Scientists are learning more and more about the microbiome daily and hope to gain a more thorough understanding of the functional interactions between us and our microbiomes in the near future, leading to new diagnostic and therapeutic capabilities.

Probiotics from food and supplements have been shown to treat and prevent diseases of the digestive tract, including diarrhea and constipation, while also treating vaginal infections, reducing the incidence of common colds and inflammatory diseases, lowering high blood pressure, preventing metabolic conditions and neurological disorders, reducing anxiety . . . the list goes on. Seriously, it's a long list!

A fantastic resource for learning more about fermented and cultured foods is *The Art of Fermentation: An In-Depth Exploration of Essential Concepts and Processes from Around the World* by Sandor Katz.

Sea Vegetables

Sea vegetables, also referred to as seaweed, are various forms of marine algae that grow naturally in coastal areas near or in saltwater. Edible seaweeds have been a staple in Asian cultures as a food and medicine for thousands of years and are growing in popularity in North America. Kombu and wakame are two popular varieties available in U.S. stores in dry packaged and fresh wet forms. Other commonly consumed algae include spirulina for smoothies and green juice, nori wrapped around sushi, and kelp noodles eaten raw.

This is an important distinction to make, considering one provides probiotics and the other does not. Most pickled foods start with a vinegar base that is typically heated to help soften and sterilize the food. Thus, fermentation is prevented by the heat and high levels of acidity from the vinegar. This means that lactic acid cannot flourish, inhibiting fermentation and the growth of beneficial bacteria or probiotics. Fermentation, as previously described, starts with various bases such as vegetable or fruit juice, water, or salt. Beneficial bacteria grow in these assorted environments with abandon and deliver many positive health outcomes. See the recipe for Lacto-Fermented Vegetables: Two Ways (page 106).

When looking for commercially fermented foods in your grocery store, make sure to read labels and find nonpasteurized versions that deliver probiotics from fermentation. Remember, heat often kills beneficial bacteria. You should find most of your fermented foods in the refrigerated section of your store, and they should contain cloudy-looking brines and/or produce small bubbles when opened.

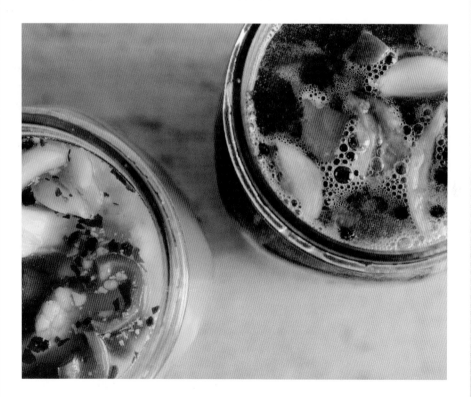

Sea vegetables offer one of the broadest ranges of minerals in any given food. Seaweed especially is a fantastic source of iron, calcium, vitamin C, and iodine. It also offers a unique mineral called vanadium, which may help to regulate carbohydrate metabolism by increasing the body's sensitivity to insulin—a good thing! Sea vegetables contain various antioxidants and have even been documented to have anti-inflammatory and antiviral capacities. Seaweed is also detoxifying due to its rich chlorophyll content, and there's promising research that shows sea vegetable consumption as a factor in lowering the risk for estrogen-related cancers like breast cancer, although more research is needed to conclude this. Check out the recipe for Vegetable Miso Soup with Kombu Dashi and Tofu (page 126), and give sea vegetables a try.

Mushrooms

Mushrooms or fungi are grown and consumed all around the world. They are considered popular and versatile forms of food and medicine. There are hundreds of edible mushrooms, including the well-known varieties we find in grocery stores. Most edible mushrooms contain protein, B vitamins, and various minerals that support a healthy immune system, and they may even reduce the risk of some forms of cancer. Some edible mushrooms can help to lower cholesterol and treat nerve disorders, while others support healthy lung function.

Mushrooms that have been exposed to sunlight outdoors or UV lamps indoors also contain vitamin D that has been shown to increase antioxidant function and brain function in humans and limit or slow microbial growth in viruses.

Science Is Cool!

Exposing many forms of edible mushrooms to direct sunlight with their gills facing up will significantly increase their vitamin D content. In one study, harvested shiitake mushrooms were exposed to the sun, gill-side up, for six hours per day for two days; researchers found that this increased vitamin D levels from 100 IU/100 grams to nearly 46,000 IU/100 grams. Vitamin D levels dropped significantly on the third day, however, due to overexposure.

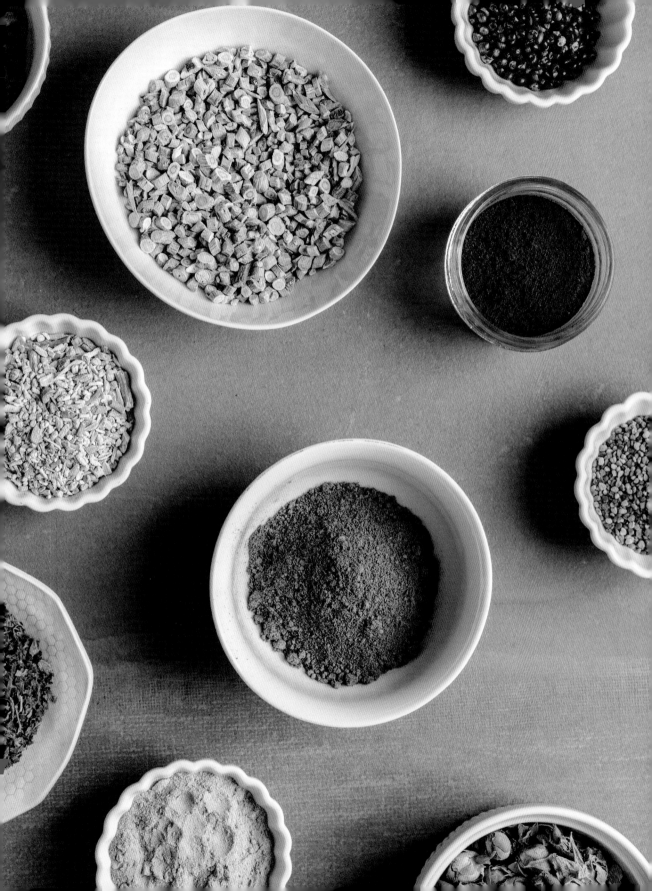

Spices and Herbs

Spices and herbs are the aromatic parts of plants that are traditionally used as medicines, fragrances, and flavorings. They have been a part of human civilization for thousands of years. Spices come from the roots, seeds, bark, and leaves of a plant, and the aroma and flavor comes mostly from their natural oils. The term *herbs* refers to the leafy greens or flowers (fresh or dried) of an herbaceous plant.

You can't talk about mushrooms, spices, and herbs without talking about adaptogens. Adaptogens are very trendy right now and for good reason. They are found in various plants, typically herbs and mushrooms, that are thought to regulate and improve stress response, decrease inflammation, and enhance immunity. Also, many, but not all, adaptogens are rich in antioxidants; one instance is chaga mushrooms, which are supposedly one of the richest sources of antioxidants found in nature. *Ashwagandha, maca,* and cordyceps are other examples of adaptogens. They typically come in powder and pill form but can also be found dried whole and in liquid tinctures. They are most effective when used as regular supplements over a period of several months rather than taken sporadically.

Certain spices and herbs have been shown to decrease pain and inflammation and even stimulate digestion. Turmeric, for example, has been studied as an anti-inflammatory agent, while black pepper has been studied as an

---

Can I Take Adaptogens while Pregnant and/or Breastfeeding?

Many of my pregnant and breastfeeding patients want to know if they can start or continue with their adaptogen intake. We are learning more about adaptogens as clinical research continues to examine their efficacy (yeah!), but unfortunately not a lot is known at this time, especially in regard to adaptogen use while pregnant and/or breastfeeding. This is the case because most parents aren't willing to use themselves or their babies as an experiment. Personally, I am not comfortable prescribing adaptogens during pregnancy or breastfeeding, as I am not a skilled or experienced herbalist, and I'm not willing to risk harm to my patients without more information. I highly recommend speaking with a trusted health professional before experimenting with them on your own, as they may interact with medications and could significantly affect your hormones while pregnant, breastfeeding, or otherwise.

Why Is Everyone Talking about Turmeric?

Turmeric deserves its own book! Turmeric is a root or rhizome, like ginger, that originates in India and dates back nearly four thousand years. It was first used as a culinary spice and in some religious ceremonies, but today it is consumed all over the world in fresh, dried, and powdered form in both food and supplements. You can find fresh turmeric in most grocery stores in the produce section near the fresh ginger. They often carry dried ground turmeric in the spice aisle as well. You can't miss it, it's bright yellow (and be warned, it stains everything!).

Curcumin is the active medicinal ingredient in turmeric, and it's known mostly for its antioxidant and anti-inflammatory properties—something from which almost everyone can benefit. Researchers are finding that it may also benefit those with inflammatory bowel disease (IBD), protect against some forms of cancer and heart disease, stimulate digestion, help to regulate blood sugar, and contribute to the prevention of Alzheimer's disease.

If you're looking for a turmeric supplement, ask your primary care physician or registered dietitian nutritionist for a recommendation. You want to find one that contains curcumin or curcuminoids, although some practitioners recommend whole turmeric extracts. Regardless, make sure you consume turmeric/curcumin, whether in food or supplements, with black pepper for increased absorption. Try the Golden Turmeric Paste recipe (page 103).

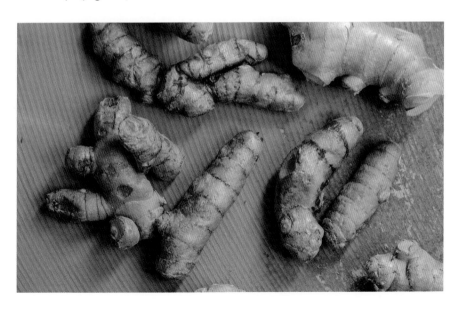

antibacterial agent as well as a compound that protects against DNA damage. Cinnamon and ginger are considered good spices to combat nausea, and rosemary is a traditional therapy used to reduce headaches. There are too many medicinal uses and health benefits of spices and herbs to name here. Two great resources for learning more about herbs and spices is *The Herbal Apothecary: 100 Medicinal Herbs and How to Use Them* by JJ Pursell, a naturopathic doctor and certified herbalist, and *The Encyclopedia of Spices and Herbs: An Essential Guide to the Flavors of the World* by Padma Lakshmi, American author and host of the cooking competition Top Chef.

Fluids

Drinking adequate noncaffeinated fluids is essential for optimal health. Water is a fantastic source and is highly recommended for daily consumption. Decaffeinated tea, milk (dairy and nondairy), unsweetened or 100 percent pure juice, and infused water are also great options for meeting your fluid needs. Consuming foods that contain water can also minimally contribute to your fluid needs.

The amount of fluid needed per person per day varies depending on age, sex, and pregnancy/breastfeeding status. Drinking adequate fluids prevents constipation, dehydration, kidney stones, moodiness, and overheating. Research shows that young adults who drink less water also drink less milk, eat fewer fruits and vegetables, drink more sugar-sweetened beverages, eat more fast food, and get less physical activity, so drink up!

The Balanced Plate

A balanced diet or plate looks different for everyone. As a registered dietitian nutritionist, it's my goal to help my patients find their unique and individualized way of eating that works best for them while considering food allergies, likes/dislikes, disease or illness, cultural preferences, family needs, and necessary nutrients for their life stage.

Depending on your chosen diet, you may or may not consume certain foods or food groups. And it must be said again, *that's OK*. You know your body best. Take care of yourself in a way that feels intuitive and good for you and your family. I offer my idea of the balanced plate for both omnivores and vegetarians/vegans, not as a rule, but as a guide. These are mere suggestions based on my research and education, but by no means are these the *right* way of eating

What If I Think I Have a Food Allergy, Sensitivity, or Intolerance?

Diagnosing a food allergy/sensitivity/intolerance can be challenging for some. Differentiating between them is an important first step. A registered dietitian nutritionist who specializes in food allergies or a board-certified allergist can help you sort out the details. First, you'll want to rule out an allergy or immune-mediated reaction that can cause life-threatening anaphylaxis.

Symptoms of a food allergy often include, but aren't limited to, itchy mouth; hives; eczema; swelling of the lips, tongue, face, or throat; wheezing; congestion; trouble breathing; gas/bloating; and nausea and/or vomiting. Typically, you'll need lab tests, a skin prick test, and whenever safe, an oral food challenge, to diagnose a food allergy.

Symptoms of a food sensitivity or intolerance include, but aren't limited to, headaches, fatigue, irritability, nausea, vomiting, stomach pain, heartburn, gas/bloating, and diarrhea. A food and symptom diary and an elimination diet that lasts two to four weeks can be helpful diagnostic tools. Also, reducing highly processed foods, sugar, and alcohol while increasing nutrient-dense foods (especially those with fiber) and fluids may improve your symptoms.

If you believe you have a food sensitivity or intolerance, work with a board-certified practitioner to help pinpoint foods that trigger adverse reactions rather than trying to self-diagnose. For many, the journey to discovering their specific food triggers can be a long one. Not knowing what makes you feel bad while having to live with persistent symptoms can be really frustrating. Ask for help and find support.

for everyone or necessarily realistic for every meal, every day. Rather, look at these guides as a place to start or a source of inspiration.

Additionally, there are many models of dietary balance. Depending on your belief system, food can be considered heating or cooling, contractive or expansive, acidic or alkalizing—various spectrums of balance you may also want to consider. You can follow different recommendations and cultural references, old or new medical perspectives, updated clinical research, or your intuition—all are valid and worthy. I believe you will have that aha moment and confidently know which diet is best for you when you find a way of eating that is realistic, sustainable, easy, and generally makes you feel good physiologically and emotionally.

Create SMART (specific, measurable, achievable, relevant, time-bound) goals to gracefully transition into a new diet or lifestyle change of any kind.

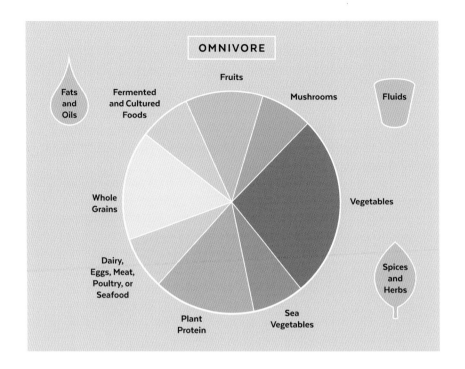

OMNIVORE

Fruits

Mushrooms

Fats and Oils

Fermented and Cultured Foods

Fluids

Whole Grains

Vegetables

Dairy, Eggs, Meat, Poultry, or Seafood

Spices and Herbs

Plant Protein

Sea Vegetables

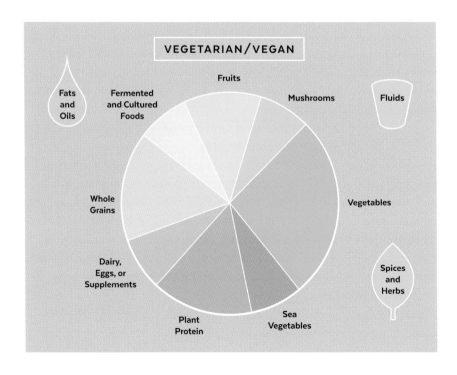

VEGETARIAN/VEGAN

Fruits

Mushrooms

Fats and Oils

Fermented and Cultured Foods

Fluids

Whole Grains

Vegetables

Dairy, Eggs, or Supplements

Spices and Herbs

Plant Protein

Sea Vegetables

If you're unsure of where to start or how, I highly encourage you to work with a trusted medical practitioner, such as a registered dietitian nutritionist, to help you sort through the details and ensure you're meeting your daily needs, especially if your diet is restrictive for any reason.

Something else to consider: Food is only one part of maintaining balance and promoting your overall health. Physical activity or body movement, as well as emotional and spiritual health, are other essential components of the bigger picture.

Body Movement

Part of a thorough nutrition assessment from a registered dietitian nutritionist includes a physical activity or body movement assessment. This can be an emotionally charged subject for some, considering that many people relate physical activity to their ability or inability to be active, their weight status, or their body image and self-worth. Research shows that negative body image is linked to poor self-care, depression, dieting, eating disorders, anxiety, substance abuse, relationship violence, and self-harm or suicide. Because of this, I believe our health care model, assessment tools, and the ways in which we approach this subject can be improved. Providers could broach this topic with more gentleness, kindness, and compassion.

Referring to physical activity or fitness as "body movement" may be more welcoming and less challenging for some, so because of this, I will refer to body movement moving forward. I believe this term also elicits a meet-you-where-you're-at attitude, being that many of us can relate to moving our bodies in some form every day versus only some of us that choose to or can partake in intense exercise or physical fitness.

There are many ways to participate in body movement. Going to the gym, running, and weight lifting are only a few of the obvious options (and disliked by so many). What I've found more effective and sustainable for my patients is to support body movement as an incorporated daily activity that allows people to have more in-depth interactions with their lives, loved ones, and surroundings. Simply put, body movement with personal value is more effective and sustainable. Many people find hiking in a beautiful gorge, stand-up paddleboarding on your favorite lake, or connecting with a friend while stretching to be more enjoyable activities than conventional gym time or regimented classes. And when we enjoy ourselves, don't you think we're more likely to try that activity again?

The current recommendations for adults from the Physical Activity Guidelines for Americans includes at least 150 to 300 minutes (2.5 to 5 hours) per week of aerobic physical activity. Additionally, muscle-strengthening activities (of moderate or greater intensity) including all major muscle groups is recommended for two or more days per week. I've created a list of alternative forms of body movement within both categories that you may find more approachable and/or relatable:

AEROBIC ACTIVITIES: yoga, hiking/backpacking, rowing, swimming, cross-country skiing, dancing, cycling, kickboxing, roller skating, power walking

MUSCLE-STRENGTHENING ACTIVITIES: gardening/digging, hiking, yoga, Pilates, rock/tree climbing, stand-up paddleboarding, kayaking, walking uphill, downhill skiing, weight-lifting

Emotional and Spiritual Health

Most of us equate the term *health* to our physical health and don't necessarily consider our emotional or mental health or our spiritual well-being. As a culture, we unfortunately don't value the mind and spirit in the same way we do the body. As integrative medicine continues to grow in popularity, this is something that will hopefully shift. I see it happening in small collectives here and there, and I wish nothing more than for Americans to see health as a holistic practice involving all aspects of self—mind, body, and spirit.

Maintaining balance in regard to our emotional health, just like eating a balanced meal, can look different for everyone. We each operate and function on different planes and need various tools to find our own personal peace. Some people feel most stable when highly functioning and productive. Others might need to prioritize "me time" more often and find a quiet space for regular personal reflection. It may take you some time, years even, to find your emotional balance.

The National Alliance on Mental Illness (NAMI) recommends the following qualities for maintaining balance: set priorities, say no, stop wasting time, plan ahead, and reflect. Can you identify one of these that you could afford to develop further? My personal favorite is saying no. As an adult, saying no can be really challenging, and it personally took me many years to develop this skill. I see now how valuable this quality is. You're actually saying yes to so much more when you say no to things that don't serve you. Give it a try!

Our spiritual health is equally as important to finding and maintaining life balance. Whether you work with intuitives and energy healers or have a traditional religious practice, spirituality is another form of self-care that needs consideration and regular fine-tuning. Practicing meditation, Reiki, or qigong; praying; journaling; going to church; participating in spiritual retreats—all are examples of opening and deepening your connection with your spirituality. When we're able to do *this* work, I believe we are able to really see what's going on within ourselves and even our surroundings and truly heal. Imagine what might be possible globally if we all prioritized this transformational work.

3
LIVING SEASONALLY

How we eat can change the world.

ALICE WATERS, CHEF, AUTHOR, FOOD ACTIVIST, AND
FOUNDER AND OWNER OF CHEZ PANISSE RESTAURANT
IN BERKELEY, CALIFORNIA

WHEREVER YOU LIVE in the world, you most likely experience some sort of seasonal variation within your local climate and environment, even if it's small. Where I live in the Pacific Northwest, I am lucky enough to observe four distinct seasons: spring, summer, autumn, and winter. And I must say, I live for the seasons, inspired by all the changes each one brings.

Sunlight, weather, temperature, food, activities, attitude, energy—there are so many variations with the coming and going of each part of the cycle. I find that if I allow myself to align with the current season, rather than ignore it or fight it, I am more relaxed and at ease, and my body feels better overall. Do you find this to be true too? Do you listen to the seasonal changes or push through them? For example, as the daylight decreases in the autumn and winter months, do you find the need to sleep more or go to bed earlier? If you allow yourself to hibernate and restore during the darker months, do you believe you will have more energy in the spring and summer months?

Just as nature rotates us through her beautiful cycles each season, our bodies have their own natural cycles called circadian rhythms that occur on a more familiar level day-to-day. Every twenty-four hours we cycle through physical, mental, and behavioral changes. Research shows that our sleep cycles, menstruation, some hormones, appetite, blood pressure, mood, digestion, body temperature, alertness, cardiovascular efficiency, and muscle strength are all influenced by this internal "season," which is regulated by the body and the external environment or exposure to sunlight, lunar cycles, and more. This innate relationship with the natural world links us to all other living beings, including plants, animals, fungi, and bacteria. Truly then, we aren't living *in* nature; we *are* nature. We are inextricably connected—woven intimately together as one.

When we override our natural rhythm, we suffer. Working night shifts long term with less exposure to sunlight, for example, has been linked to increased chronic diseases and illnesses, such as heart disease, gastrointestinal issues, weight gain, obesity, irregular eating habits, depression, and more. Or when we don't honor the seasonal changes in our food system, both in farming practices and our diets, the environment suffers, and we can become sluggish and energetically stagnant. When we choose to live in the flow with nature and holistically support our health and happiness, we can thrive.

Aligning with the Seasons

Just as nature slowly walks her way into each season, you too want to transition gracefully—always striving for a gentle balance rather than harsh extremes. Try to look at your habits and qualities from a bird's-eye view, where you can see the whole picture, and notice general trends rather than focusing on only one area. This can be hard to do at times, so seek counsel and support when needed.

I've created a chart that highlights various seasonal qualities from multiple perspectives I've studied along my journey. This can act as an investigative tool to help you better understand the intuitive and seasonal changes in nature while also learning more about your own personal climate. You may recognize your unique constitution in this chart as it relates to one or many seasons. Do you have slow digestion? Do you need a lot of sleep? Do you crave salty foods? Certain qualities will be easier to identify than others. Become curious and pay attention. Listen. Eventually, with time and intention, a deeper understanding will unveil itself.

QUESTIONS TO CONSIDER

- Which season are you?

- Which season(s) do you relate to the most? Which quality is the most resonant?

- Are you aligned with the current season?

- Do your physiological, digestive, and emotional qualities change with each season? Does one aspect change more than the others?

- Which of your qualities needs the most shifting to align with the current season?

	SPRING	SUMMER	AUTUMN	WINTER
Physiological	Increasing energy	Increasing energy	Decreasing energy	Decreasing energy
	Less sleep needed	Less sleep needed	More sleep needed	More sleep needed
	Less heat produced	Less heat produced	More heat produced	More heat produced
	Increasing metabolism	Increasing metabolism	Decreasing metabolism	Decreasing metabolism
	Weight loss	Weight loss	Weight gain	Weight gain
	Increasing immunity	Increasing immunity	Decreasing immunity	Decreasing immunity
	Increasing allergies/ asthma	Increasing inflammation/ injury	Increasing viral infections	Increasing viral infections
	Decreasing sex drive	Decreasing sex drive	Increasing sex drive	Increasing sex drive
Digestive	Decreasing appetite	Decreasing appetite	Increasing appetite	Increasing appetite
	Faster digestion	Faster digestion	Slower digestion	Slower digestion
	Increasing insulin resistance	Decreasing insulin resistance	Increasing insulin resistance	Increasing insulin resistance
	More frequent, smaller meals	More frequent, smaller meals	Less frequent, larger meals	Less frequent, larger meals
	Detoxification			
Macro- nutrients	Decrease protein	Decrease protein	Increase protein	Increase protein
	Decrease fats	Decrease fats	Increase fats	Increase fats
	Decrease carbohydrates	Decrease carbohydrates	Increase carbohydrates	Increase carbohydrates
Food Groups*	Plant-based protein	Plant-based protein	Animal protein	Animal protein
	Fresh vegetables	Fresh vegetables	Starchy vegetables	Starchy vegetables
	Delicate greens/ sprouts	Delicate greens/ sprouts	Cooked vegetables	Cooked vegetables
	Whole grains	Whole grains	Hearty greens	Hearty greens
	Fruits	Fruits	Whole grains	Whole grains
	Dairy	Dairy	Fruits	Fruits
	Mushrooms	Mushrooms	Mushrooms	
	Edible flowers	Sea vegetables	Sea vegetables	
		Edible flowers		
Emotional	Insightful	Expressive	Reflective	Contemplative
	Ambivert	Extrovert	Ambivert	Introvert
	More vocal	Vocal	More quiet	Quiet
	More excitable	Excited	More calm	Calm
	Renewed	Empowered	Released	Surrendered
	Decreased stress/ anxiety	Decreased stress/ anxiety	Increased stress/ anxiety	Increased stress/ anxiety

* See Appendix A for seasonal produce chart

→

	SPRING	SUMMER	AUTUMN	WINTER
Traditional Chinese Medicine	Sour Cooling Expansive Yin	Bitter Cooling Sweet (late summer) Neutral to warming (late summer) Expansive (late summer) Yang (late summer)	Pungent Warming or cooling Contractive Yang	Salty Cooling Contractive Yin
Ayurveda	Pungent Bitter Astringent Cool Damp/moist Heavy Oily Slow Stable Sinus/chest congestion Sluggish digestion Lethargy Sadness	Sweet Bitter Astringent Hot Humid Sharp Bright Humid Acne Inflammation Acidic stomach Irritability	Sweet Bitter Astringent Cool Dry Light Rough Windy Clear Itching Dry eyes Loose stools Unstable emotions	Sweet Sour Salty Cold Dry Hard Clear Stiff joints Weight gain Constipation Anxiety
Cooking Techniques	Fry Steam Sauté Blanch/poach Raw/fresh	Grill Steam Sauté Blanch/poach Raw/fresh Preserve/ferment Batch cook	Grill Bake Roast Slow cook/stew Preserve/ferment Batch cook	Fry Bake Roast Slow cook/stew
Body Movement	Stretching Jogging Kundalini or Iyengar yoga Hiking Cycling Gardening Tai chi Qigong Pilates	Stretching Running Hatha or Vinyasa yoga Hiking Cycling Gardening Swimming Tai chi Qigong Pilates	Stretching Jogging Kundalini or Iyengar yoga Hiking Tai chi Qigong Pilates	Stretching Walking Restorative yoga Tai chi Qigong Pilates

Please note that this chart is not saying that you can't dance in the winter or eat starchy vegetables in the summer. Rather, it offers you a way of living and eating that allows you to align more holistically with nature and the energetic rhythms surrounding you. Allowing the seasons to guide us can translate to more balance, health, and harmony within ourselves.

Once you've clearly identified your seasonal constitution, you may notice that another season offers you challenges. If you're a summer person, for example, who doesn't need a lot of sleep, eats small meals throughout the day comprised mostly of fresh produce and plant proteins, and loves high-intensity workouts, you may find that winter is challenging for you. These qualities don't flow as easily in the winter months. If you can offer yourself more time to sleep, you may notice that your energy level shifts and feels adequate. You eat larger meals less often of roasted vegetables, stewed meats, and hearty whole grains; and your digestion and hunger/fullness feel balanced. You change your style of body movement to something more restorative to suit the slower pace of winter, and your body feels resilient and rested.

When looking to make change(s), remember to start small. A stellar way to begin the shift toward more seasonal living is to choose one category or subcategory from the Seasonal Qualities chart and start there. I like to recommend starting with seasonal foods and cooking techniques. Of course, I recommend starting with your food—I'm a registered dietitian nutritionist! When you move closer to eating a seasonal diet, not only will you feel a significant difference in your body and overall mood, but you will also experience so many other benefits. Refer to the seasonal recipes in Chapters 5 through 9 for deeper inspiration.

As a reminder, these are some of the benefits of seasonal eating, as described more thoroughly in Chapter 1:

- Better texture, flavor, and color of foods

- More nutrition bite for bite

- Better support of seasonal health needs

- Less toxic chemical exposure

- Preservation of natural resources and lower environmental impact

- Money saving

- Support for your local food economy

Intuitive Medicine

In my opinion, one of our best tools for improving our health is learning to identify and listen to our inner voice, especially in regard to diet and nutrition. This is what I call intuitive medicine. I strongly encourage you to find the voice inside yourself, if you haven't already. This even pertains to my Seasonal Qualities chart. Listen to what your inner voice is telling you about it. If you don't connect with my approach or perspective, then find another resource with which you do connect.

Case Studies

A sixty-year-old woman came to me to try to figure out why she was always hungry—and thus always eating. She also complained of severe fatigue. She ate multiple meals and snacks comprised mostly of whole foods daily, but she could never seem to reach satiety. After further assessment, including lab work and coordination of care with her primary care physician, we ruled out any major deficiencies and illnesses. We identified her personality and constitution as one that's split between the spring and summer seasons. She reported that she rarely ate starchy vegetables or whole grains and, in general, had a low carbohydrate intake. In the spring and summer months, this didn't seem to affect her as much, but it did in the autumn and winter. We worked together to find creative ways for her to increase those food groups, especially during the colder weather. After some time, she reported that this slight adjustment made a big difference with her satiety and also provided her with more energy, which she said was a blessing, because she had been starting to believe that she was just supposed to feel tired as she aged.

I had another patient come to me for help with her digestive issues. She was a twenty-eight-year-old woman who identified herself as someone who thrives in the cooler winter months. At the time of this appointment (midsummer), she was battling daily low gastrointestinal pain, especially after eating, and constipation. She was also unintentionally gaining weight. After reviewing her chart, consulting with her primary care physician and ruling out more serious GI problems, as well as reviewing her diet recall, I noticed she typically ate two or three large meals a day. As a starting place, I recommended that she try eating five or six smaller meals or larger snacks instead and focus on fresh seasonal vegetables and fruits. This recommendation wasn't invasive or even that big of a shift for her since she loved fresh produce and had a beautiful garden, and it was just what she needed. Her lower GI pain decreased dramatically in a few short weeks, and she began having regular bowel movements with little effort. For her, this was a good reminder that her diet is flexible and needed to shift with the seasons to better meet her digestive needs.

You will get medical and health advice from a variety of people, most of it well intentioned but not always in line with your true inner wisdom or self-care goals. You may become conflicted when this happens because "an expert" is telling you how to change something, how to prevent or heal an illness, how to live a certain lifestyle. Maybe your personal views don't align with the advice, or maybe you can't pinpoint why, but something inside you doesn't resonate with it—something doesn't feel right. *Listen to that inner voice.* Above everything else, your inner voice and intuition are your best guide.

I hear stories from my patients all the time. Your doctor or someone on your health care team tells you that you need to do something like calorie count daily, lose a certain amount of weight, start an extremely restrictive diet (sadly, I hear this one far too often), or avoid a specific food group altogether. Whatever it is, it's a recommendation that doesn't feel right or sit well with you. Maybe you even go as far as to try the said recommendation, adopt the new diet, take the diet pills, before realizing it's not what you want. Or maybe you are lucky enough to hear your inner voice telling you "no thanks" before you even go down that road. My point is, although intangible and unseen, your intuition is worthy. *You* are worthy. You may doubt yourself and your "qualifications" or credentials, but somewhere deep inside, you know what you need and don't need!

Remember, you hold the power. You are the owner of your healing process. This does not mean you should self-diagnose or self-prescribe supplements or diets, but you need to move your opinion and your intuition to the top of the decision ladder. Because, truly, nobody knows you better than you know yourself. Nobody knows what you need better than you do. When we trust ourselves and allow ourselves to relax in this empowered space, the answers will be much easier to see. So when a trusted source suggests a therapeutic approach and it sounds intuitive, sustainable, and balanced and generally makes you feel good, listen to that and proceed accordingly.

After further consideration, if your path still appears foggy and you're unsure of what you need or where to begin regarding food, nutrition, diet, or body movement, I highly recommend working in person with a registered dietitian nutritionist. Do your research and find someone with credentials who supports your beliefs. I recommend working with someone who approaches food and nutrition from an integrative and functional medicine (IFM) perspective. These practitioners look at *how* and *why* illness or disease occurs and address the root cause while treating the individual with evidence-based medicine. I also recommend a non-diet or anti-diet registered dietitian nutritionist who supports intuitive eating or mindful eating concepts.

4

AT HOME IN YOUR KITCHEN

We can change the way we make and get our food so that it becomes food again—something that feeds our bodies and our souls. Imagine it: Every meal would connect us to the joy of living and the wonder of nature. Every meal would be like saying grace.

MICHAEL POLLAN, AMERICAN AUTHOR, JOURNALIST, ACTIVIST, AND PROFESSOR AT HARVARD UNIVERSITY AND UC BERKELEY

CREATING A WHOLE FOODS pantry is quite simple, and it will pay off tenfold in the long run. If you have an existing food pantry, allow yourself time to slowly transition from your current stock to more nutritious, whole foods by replacing one pantry category at a time. If you don't already keep a pantry, use this chapter to help you establish one.

Keeping a well-stocked whole foods pantry will make cooking a balanced diet more easily attainable and effortlessly sustainable. You will have what you need for those last-minute meals or snacks and for the ones you plan ahead too. You will also save money and time. Buying in bulk is one way you can save money (typically) and extend the benefits of your pantry. Other ways include saving your food scraps to create flavorful broths and stocks, batch cooking (see page 116), and freezing previously cooked foods and premade meals.

Make Homemade Stock

Keep a glass container or freezer bag in your freezer and add food scraps (including bones, organs, shells, vegetable ends, peels, stems, and so on) as you accumulate them. Once the container is full, make a delicious homemade stock by covering the ingredients with water in a stockpot and bringing them to a gentle boil, then simmering for at least 1 hour. If you're feeling really organized and have the space, designate different freezer containers for different types of stock. Consider separating vegetables, bones and animal parts, and seafood scraps and shells into three individual containers for vegetable, chicken and/or beef, and seafood stock.

Maintaining a whole foods pantry can also benefit the environment. Food production is the single biggest cause of deforestation, and decomposing wasted food is one of the largest contributors to greenhouse gas emissions. Annually, 40 percent of food produced in the U.S. goes to waste—that's more than a billion pounds of food every year! Learning to properly store food will not only help it last longer, but it will also contribute to reducing overall food waste and global warming.

Compost

Whether you participate in your city's local composting program or personally maintain a compost heap for your home garden or yard, you are positively contributing to the health of the global community. According to the Environmental Protection Agency, composting food waste keeps unnecessary decomposing food out of landfills, enriches soil, reduces the need for chemical fertilizers on a small and large scale, minimizes water usage, and decreases greenhouse gas emissions while lowering your carbon footprint.

Food Storage

If you're willing to invest time and intention into maintaining a whole foods diet, then you need to set aside time to adequately prepare for food and pantry storage as well. This may seem like an afterthought or a small detail, but without the necessary food storage equipment, creating and sustaining a whole foods pantry—or diet, for that matter—will be challenging.

I recommend using glass containers exclusively, whether you purchase new glassware or assemble a collection from different sources. I use a

 The average person throws away 185 pounds of plastic every year, and 91 percent of total recyclable plastic is actually not recycled. If you must use plastic containers, be sure to look for the number inside the small triangle on your container. Each number indicates which type of resin or plastic is used. Avoid numbers 3, 6, and 7 as these plastics may contain bisphenol A (BPA), which has been found to be an endocrine (hormone) disruptor. Research shows it increases the risk for female and male infertility, abnormal advanced puberty, hormone-dependent tumors, breast and prostate cancer, and metabolic disorders such as polycystic ovary syndrome (PCOS).

combination of glass jars and glass food storage containers with screw-on and snap-on lids in various sizes for my pantry. I prefer glass to plastic because plastic food storage containers, including those made of BPA-free plastics, can leach dangerous chemicals into your food and may pose a health risk, especially when heated or storing liquids. Plastic containers are also a hazard for the environment and contribute to greenhouse gas emissions. Alternatives to plastic include glass, cloth, beeswax products, and stainless steel.

Consider labeling your pantry items to use your ingredients most efficiently. Waterproof labels are also helpful, so you can wash your containers easily without having to remove the labels or create new ones.

Here are some other helpful techniques for keeping a whole foods pantry:

- Meal plan and menu plan before shopping and stocking your pantry.

- Schedule weekly meal prep time (such as every Sunday afternoon from 2:00 to 4:00).

- Batch cook (cook once for multiple meals/snacks).

- Use proper storage containers. Do you have what you need?

- Leave yourself friendly reminders for restocking items and new ingredients (sticky notes, calendar reminders, chalkboard list, etc.).

- Stay flexible! Even small changes take time.

Now that you've spent time organizing your pantry, don't let your precious ingredients spoil. Know which food items should be stored in your pantry versus in the refrigerator or freezer.

PANTRY	REFRIGERATOR OR FREEZER
Whole grains	Whole-grain flours, sprouted whole grains
Beans and legumes	Dairy, eggs, meat, and poultry
Dried sea vegetables	Seafood
Oils (most)	Fresh sea vegetables
Spices and dried herbs	Nuts and seeds (freezer)
Canned, jarred, and nonperishable items	Flax oil, flavored oils
Dried mushrooms	Fresh herbs
Vinegars	Fermented and cultured foods
Sweeteners	Fresh mushrooms

Pantry Essentials

I've included a list of recommended ingredients for each food category in this section. Consider this a starting place—not a complete list. These recommendations are based on *my* preferences while considering quality, accessibility, nutritional content, and sustainability. Each category also includes helpful information about storage, as well as food preparation and cooking tips.

Fruits

Apples, avocados, bananas, blueberries, cranberries, dates, lemons, limes, oranges, peaches, pears, strawberries, tomatoes

Fruit is full of natural sugar (yum!) and many beneficial nutrients and antioxidants. Choose seasonal fruits whenever possible for optimal flavor and vitamin and mineral content. Refer to the Environmental Working Group's Dirty Dozen and Clean Fifteen lists for when to prioritize organic versus nonorganic (read more about this in Chapter 1).

STORAGE. Don't clean your fruit before storing. Washing your fruit adds moisture, which encourages bacterial growth and may cause faster spoilage. Store your fruit separately, especially your bananas, from other produce since they emit ethylene gas that can prematurely ripen and spoil other produce. Once your fruit has reached the desired ripeness, keep it in the refrigerator to stall further ripening.

PREPARATION/COOKING. Fresh, frozen, dried, or 100 percent juice are all great fruit options, but remember that fruit juice does not contain the beneficial fiber that whole fruit does, so try to consume fruit in its whole form whenever possible. Raw or cooked preparations are both fantastic ways to enjoy fruit. Consider peeling all nonorganic fruits before eating to minimize your exposure to toxic chemicals.

Go Bananas!

Next time you buy bananas, buy two bunches—one for eating fresh and one for freezing. This way you'll always have some on hand for smoothies and frozen desserts, such as the Strawberry Vanilla Almond Butter Smoothie with Bee Pollen (page 121).

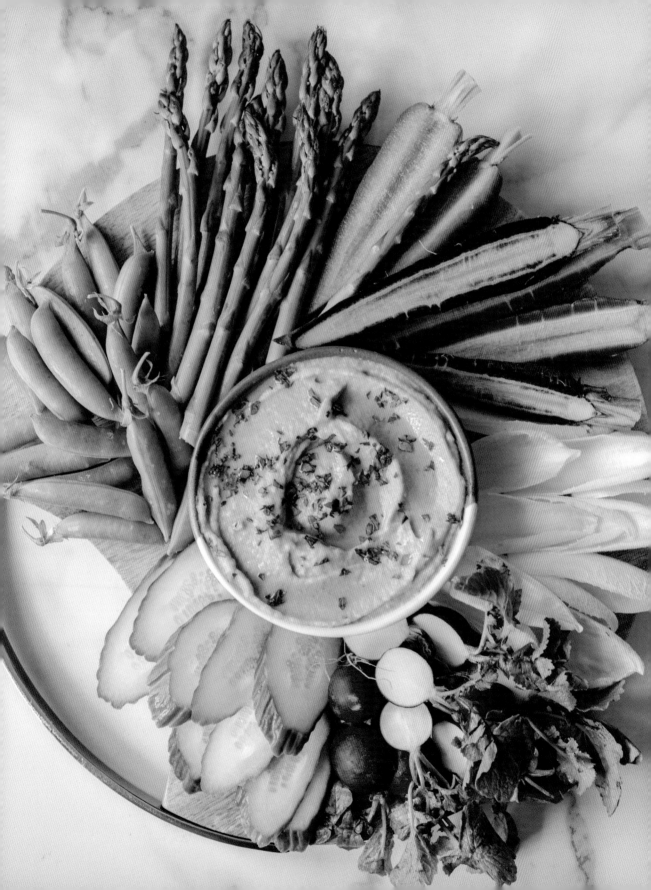

Vegetables

Cruciferous vegetables (broccoli, bok choy, brussel sprouts, cabbage, cauliflower, radishes); leafy greens (kale, red leaf lettuce, spinach, swiss chard); starchy vegetables (beets, squash, sweet potatoes, yams); carrots; celery; garlic; onions; sprouts

Vegetables deliver so many important nutrients and, sadly, are often missing from American plates. Actually, one-third of all vegetables consumed in the U.S. come from potato chips, iceberg lettuce, and French fries. Choose seasonal vegetables whenever possible, and remember to eat a variety of rainbow-colored vegetables to ensure a healthy and diverse dose of vitamins and minerals in your diet. Refer to the Environmental Working Group's Dirty Dozen and Clean Fifteen lists to learn more about when to buy organic versus nonorganic vegetables (refer to Chapter 1).

STORAGE. Don't clean your vegetables before storing them. Just like with fruit, washing your vegetables adds moisture, which encourages bacterial growth and may cause faster spoilage. Store your vegetables in a reusable and breathable mesh bag in the refrigerator for proper air circulation and to prolong shelf life and avoid the overuse of plastic bags.

PREPARATION/COOKING. Consider eating a variety of raw and cooked vegetables to ensure you're consuming a wide range of nutrients and enzymes. Consider peeling all nonorganic vegetables before eating to minimize your exposure to toxic chemicals. Fresh, frozen, dried, or 100 percent juice are all respectable forms. If you're making vegetable juice, try to find a use for the pulp too (Veggie burgers? Add into baked goods?), since it contains so much beneficial fiber.

Whole Grains

Short- and long-grain brown rice, polenta (corn grits), masa harina (corn flour), quinoa, rolled oats, wild rice, wheat berries, whole grain bread, whole grain or corn tortillas, whole wheat pasta

Choose whole grains over refined grains whenever possible for optimal protein content, fiber, B vitamins, and other valuable nutrients. Purchase organic grains, especially on high-yield grain crops like wheat, to ensure you have a food product that was grown and harvested without toxic chemicals and that contains maximum nutrients.

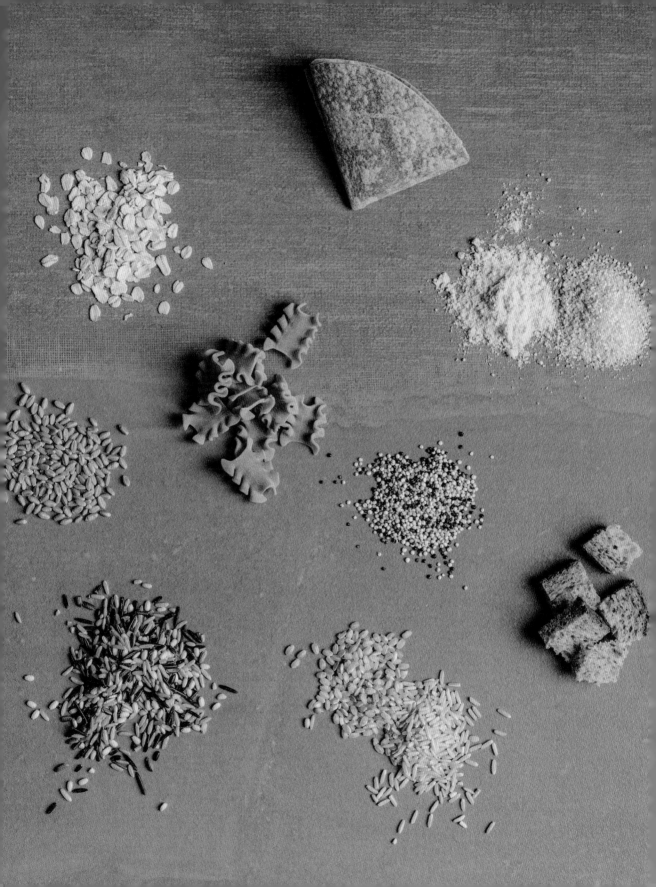

STORAGE. You can store whole grains in your pantry in an airtight container. If you're using sprouted whole grains, you must keep them in your refrigerator or freezer. Keep whole grain flours, sprouted or not, in the refrigerator or freezer for a longer shelf life, especially if you're purchasing in large quantities.

PREPARATION/COOKING. Consider soaking your whole grains in water for at least 8 hours or overnight before cooking to speed up the cooking time and to increase digestibility by neutralizing the phytic acid content. Soaking will also activate the plant embryo, a process known as "sprouting," which will deliver more available nutrients than mature nonsprouted grains. Consider buying sprouted whole grains and whole grain flours if you're unable to soak your grains first.

Eggs, Dairy, Meat, and Poultry

Beef, cultured butter, butter, buttermilk, chicken, chicken eggs, cow's milk, goat/ sheep cheese, kefir, Parmesan cheese, whole milk sour cream, whole milk yogurt

Look for high-quality, USDA organic, grass-fed or pastured, free-range, certified humane animal products. Yes, this is quite a list but such an important one (refer to Chapter 1, page 12 for more information). If you're unable to find or afford animal products with these qualifications, consider buying these foods from small local farms where you can personally verify quality farming practices and animal welfare without the often pricey and formal certifications. Also, consider shopping at grocery stores that have their own animal product rating system for quality food.

STORAGE. Store all commercial eggs in your refrigerator. If your eggs are farm fresh and have not been washed or pasteurized, you can safely store them at room temperature for two weeks or refrigerated for three months. Dairy, meat, and poultry need to be stored in the refrigerator or freezer and used by the "Best By" date on the packaging (or when your sight, smell, and common sense inform you).

PREPARATION/COOKING. In general, the longer animal products are cooked, the more nutrients they lose. Consider less lengthy cooking methods like boiling and sautéing versus stewing to preserve more nutrition. Follow food safety guidelines whenever possible, and consider using a meat thermometer to measure desired doneness temperature.

Seafood

Clams, cod, crab, lobster, mussels, oysters, prawns, salmon, scallops, tilapia, trout, tuna

Always choose sustainable seafood. In general, pole, troll, and line-caught wild seafood is optimal unless overfished in your area, and then farmed seafood is recommended. Both wild and farmed seafood can have severe and negative impacts on our environment and marine life population. Know when to prioritize wild versus farmed seafood and what to look for, as there are many ways to harvest seafood in the wild and on farms. Not all ways are created equal.

STORAGE. Prioritize fresh or "frozen at sea," sometimes called "fresh-frozen," seafood for the best flavor. If storing fresh fish, refrigerate and use within one or two days for optimal freshness. Shellfish should be purchased live and placed in a shallow pan or bowl, covered with a moistened towel, and refrigerated for two to three days (clams and mussels) or up to ten days (oysters). Live crabs or lobsters should be cooked the same day they're purchased. Fish and shucked shellfish can be frozen, although it's best to buy frozen seafood directly from the source since suppliers have better freezing methods that ensure the highest quality and safety.

PREPARATION/COOKING. There are many fantastic ways to prepare seafood. Seafood tends to be more delicate and needs less cooking time than meat or poultry, so consider more gentle methods like sautéing, steaming, or poaching. Fish will become opaque and firm when cooked, and shellfish will open their shells when ready. Follow food safety recommendations for cooking seafood to avoid foodborne illness.

Monterey Bay Seafood Watch Consumer Guide

Use this amazing *free* resource for updated sustainability and fishing/farming information specific to your area. The app and website, including the Consumer's Guide, offer clear recommendations with helpful categories (best choices, good alternatives, avoid) to make eating out and buying sustainable seafood easy and convenient.

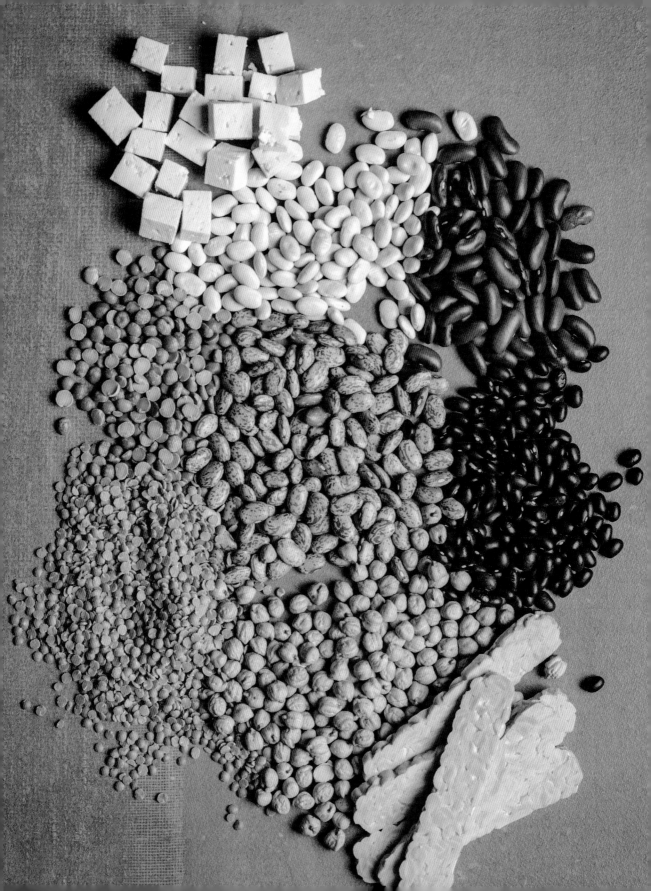

Beans and Legumes

Black beans, chickpeas (garbanzo beans), kidney beans, lentils, pinto beans, soybeans (tofu, tempeh), white beans (cannellini, Great Northern, corona)

Beans and legumes are loaded with valuable nutrients and fiber. In general, I recommend prioritizing plant-based proteins, such as beans and legumes, while minimizing animal protein whenever possible. Buy dried beans and legumes versus canned for better quality and flavor, and to avoid unnecessary additives (although a can of beans may just save a weeknight dinner!).

STORAGE. Store your dried beans and legumes in airtight jars in your dry pantry along with your canned beans. Dry beans and legumes will last for many years, although for the best quality and faster cooking time, consume them within one year of the purchase date. Vitamin degradation is thought to occur after two to three years of storage.

PREPARATION/COOKING. Beans are super versatile. Although they can take some time to cook (compared to canned beans), in my opinion, they're worth every minute. They easily adopt the flavors of other ingredients used in preparation and cooking, especially when you cook dried beans traditionally on the stovetop with vegetable, chicken, or beef stock instead of water. I also like to use a pressure cooker for dried beans to speed up the cooking time and infuse more flavor.

According to America's Test Kitchen, brining beans in a salt solution overnight can also create a more tender, smoother consistency, while contributing to the health benefits of overnight soaking (reduced gas and increased digestibility). If you're using canned beans, discard the liquid and thoroughly rinse the beans before eating to help reduce gas.

Nuts and Seeds

Almonds (butter, flour, whole nuts), cashews (butter, whole nuts), chia seeds, flaxseeds, hemp seeds, pecans, pistachios, pumpkin seeds, sesame seeds (paste, whole seeds), sunflower seeds, walnuts

Choose raw, organic, shelled nuts whenever possible or conventionally grown nuts in the shell to avoid unwanted toxins. Read ingredient labels carefully, as many are coated with salt, flavorings, and preservatives before they're packaged. As for seeds, look for unhulled or whole seeds that include all of their original parts, whenever possible, for higher nutrient content and a less adulterated food.

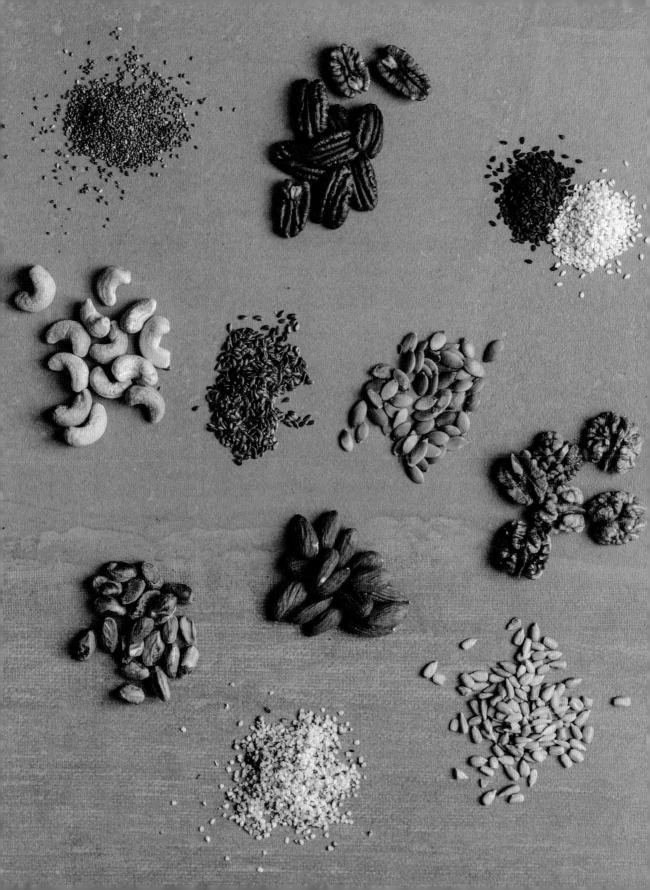

STORAGE. Store all nuts and seeds in airtight containers in the freezer for up to one year to maintain optimal nutrition and flavor. Small quantities can be stored in your dry pantry if you plan to use them sooner rather than later. Home-roasted nuts should be consumed within a short time to preserve the highest nutrient composition.

PREPARATION/COOKING. The most nutrient-rich form of nuts and seeds is raw. However, flavor and aroma will increase when you dry roast them. Whenever you can, dry roast, candy, and/or season your nuts and seeds yourself to preserve the most nutrition and avoid the unwanted ingredients in commercial preparations. Research shows that dry roasting between 160°F and 300°F for 10 to 20 minutes preserves the most nutrients in nuts and seeds, although flaxseeds and walnuts are most nutritious when eaten raw.

Fats and Oils

Cultured butter, pastured butter, cold-pressed unrefined coconut oil, cold-pressed extra virgin olive oil, cold-pressed flaxseed oil, ghee, unrefined toasted sesame oil

Choose solid or saturated fats like butter and coconut oil from grassfed animals, USDA organic, and sustainable sources. Look for unrefined and expeller-pressed or cold-pressed unsaturated oils whenever possible. Use refined expeller-pressed oils (grapeseed, sunflower, peanut, and so on) sparingly, if at all; the processing methods used are potentially harmful and toxic.

STORAGE. Store your butter in the refrigerator for longer shelf life or at room temperature if you will consume it within one to two weeks. Flaxseed oil and

What's the Best Way to Consume Flaxseeds—Whole, Ground, or Oil?

Flaxseeds are high in fiber and healthy fats (omega-3 fatty acids). They also contain beneficial phytonutrients such as lignans, which may prevent hormone-associated cancers, osteoporosis, and cardiovascular disease. Ground flaxseeds (flaxseed meal) are the optimal way to consume flax because the whole form often passes through your intestines undigested, and flaxseed oil doesn't contain the beneficial phytoestrogens of the seed. You can buy ground flaxseeds or grind your own whole seeds in a coffee grinder or food processor.

flavored oils that are used less often should be stored in your refrigerator. Coconut, olive, and sesame oil and ghee can be kept in a dry, cool, dark place such as your pantry. Keep all oil out of direct sunlight. Store all of your oils in dark-colored glass bottles, or cover the bottles with foil or another opaque material to minimize light exposure.

PREPARATION/COOKING. Each fat and oil has its own distinct flavor and function. Consider using different fats and oils for different culinary techniques. Each has a unique smoke point (the temperature at which it will literally begin to smoke), which will inevitably limit its uses. Once this happens, the beneficial fats will degrade and cause your oil to get bitter, to burn, and even to catch fire. In general, remember that the higher the smoke point, the more cooking methods you can use it for. Olive oil, for example, has a fairly low smoke point of 325°F to 375°F and is best used for low-temperature sautéing or in a dressing that does not require heat. Ghee has a high smoke point of 485°F and can be used for higher temperature cooking methods like frying or searing. Learn how to make your own Ghee on page 101.

Fermented and Cultured Foods
Kimchi, miso, olives, pickles, sauerkraut, shoyu or tamari

Fermentation is a form of food preservation that boosts nutritional value. It's a natural phenomenon where microbes in the air inoculate or culture a food through an anaerobic process. Nowadays, cultures are added to most commercially fermented foods to help start the fermentation process, control the potency, and save time. When purchasing fermented or cultured foods, choose refrigerated, unpasteurized versions and look for the words *fermented* or *naturally fermented* on the packaging. Keep in mind that if a food is heat-treated (pasteurized, fried, and so on), the probiotic-rich organisms are decreased or inactivated depending on temperature and time. Look for bubbles when you open a jar or container of fermented or cultured food—a telltale sign of fermentation. Better yet, make fermented and cultured foods yourself at home to ensure the utmost health properties and potency. Check out Lacto-Fermented Vegetables: Two Ways and Plain Whole Milk Yogurt on pages 106 and 110 for inspiration.

STORAGE. Store-bought ferments should be kept in the refrigerator. Home-made ferments can be kept at room temperature while processing, but they

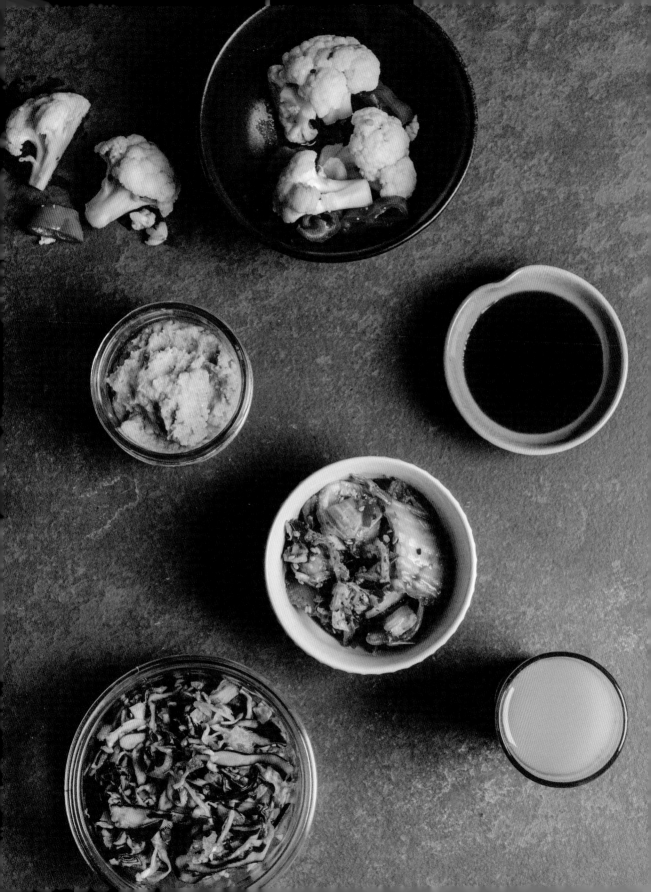

will continue to ferment over time, making the end product more sour and sometimes "spicier." When you've reached optimal flavor and stage of fermentation, you can opt to put your ferments in the refrigerator or a dry, cold pantry space like a cellar or garage to stall the fermentation process.

PREPARATION/COOKING. Making fermented and cultured foods is easy and fun! These foods are often eaten raw since cooking or heating can damage the probiotic content. However, researchers are finding that after baking, the probiotic bacteria in sourdough bread recovers and actually continues to populate. It's exciting to think about what other baked or heated ferments might survive after heating. Injera (Ethiopian flatbread), buttermilk pancakes?! Also, do you remember the difference between pickling and fermenting or culturing food? This is an important differentiation to keep in mind when in the kitchen. Read more about this on page 46.

Sea Vegetables
Blue-green algae, dulse, kombu, nori, wakame

Seaweed is incredibly nutritious and diverse—truly a superfood. Always choose sustainably harvested seaweed. Wild seaweed is preferred over farmed seaweed, as long as it's sourced from clean waters. Also, buy locally sourced seaweed, if possible, to support your local economy and guarantee the freshest product with the shortest distance traveled.

STORAGE. You can store fresh or living seaweed in a solution of table salt and sterile water (like ocean water) and refrigerate for four to seven days, depending on the quality. Dried seaweed should be stored in airtight containers in your pantry where it will last for several years. Any exposure to moisture can be managed by redehydrating it in your oven or dehydrator.

PREPARATION/COOKING. Fresh seaweed pairs well with soups and stews, salads, smoothies, marinades, and more, adding a salty, "green," umami flavor. Dried seaweed can be ground or finely chopped and used in a shaker or reconstituted in water and then added to a recipe as a salt alternative or natural seasoning. Although lacking strong research to support it, one recommendation for preserving the most nutrients is to add your fresh or dried seaweed toward the end of cooking time to expose it to less heat.

What Is a Superfood?

Superfoods are nutrient-dense foods that provide a multitude of health benefits. The term *superfood* doesn't actually come with standard criteria or a qualifying list of foods; rather, it is a fun word to use for foods that pack an extra nutritional punch. Superfoods are usually made up of colorful, unprocessed, whole foods like blueberries, salmon, seaweed, and spinach. They contain macro- and micronutrients and various other constituents that have many different health benefits for your body.

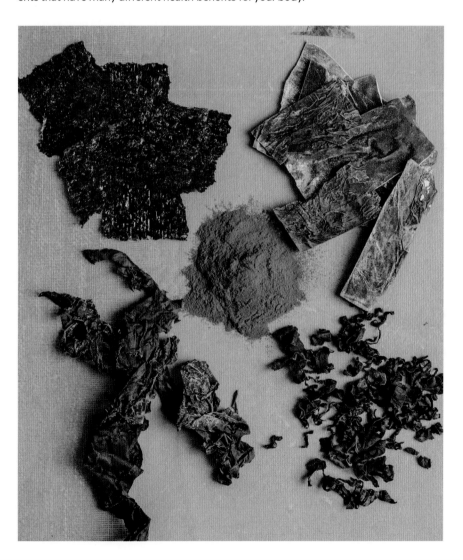

Mushrooms

Chanterelles, enoki, morels, oyster, porcini, shiitake

As culinary and medicinal mushrooms become more popular in the U.S., more varieties are being cultivated, harvested, and readily found at grocery stores and farmer's markets. They offer a wide range of nutrients and flavors, providing earthy substance and umami to any dish. Make sure to always choose ethically harvested mushrooms, or harvest your own if you feel confident identifying the edible varieties.

STORAGE. You can purchase fresh or dried mushrooms at most grocery stores and farmer's markets. Fresh packaged mushrooms should be left in their packaging and refrigerated until you are ready to use them. When buying bulk mushrooms, place them in a reusable container and wrap tightly with plastic wrap, mimicking commercial packaging. This method will keep your mushrooms fresh for about one week. If you're buying dried mushrooms, remove them from their original packaging and store them in an airtight container; keep them in a dry pantry until you're ready to use them. Properly stored dried mushrooms should last for several years.

PREPARATION/COOKING. Clean your fresh mushrooms using a damp paper towel. Do not submerge them in water or they will retain extra moisture, and their texture will become gummy and soggy. Some physicians strongly advise against eating raw mushrooms of any kind, speculating that they contain a natural carcinogen. Although more research is needed to substantiate this claim, I would err on the side of caution and avoid eating them raw. Sautéing, broiling, or adding them to your favorite soups are all great options.

Herbs and Spices

Black pepper (whole peppercorns, ground), cayenne, chai, chives (fresh, dried), cinnamon (sticks, ground), coriander (seeds, ground), garlic (fresh, powder), ginger (fresh, ground), oregano (fresh, dried), parsley (fresh, dried), red pepper flakes, thyme (fresh, dried), turmeric (fresh, ground)

Herbs and spices elevate and transform any dish. Consider purchasing your dried spices and herbs from a specialty spice store rather than your local grocery store for optimal quality and reduced prices. Also, consider growing herbs at home and drying them yourself for ultimate freshness. Buy dried

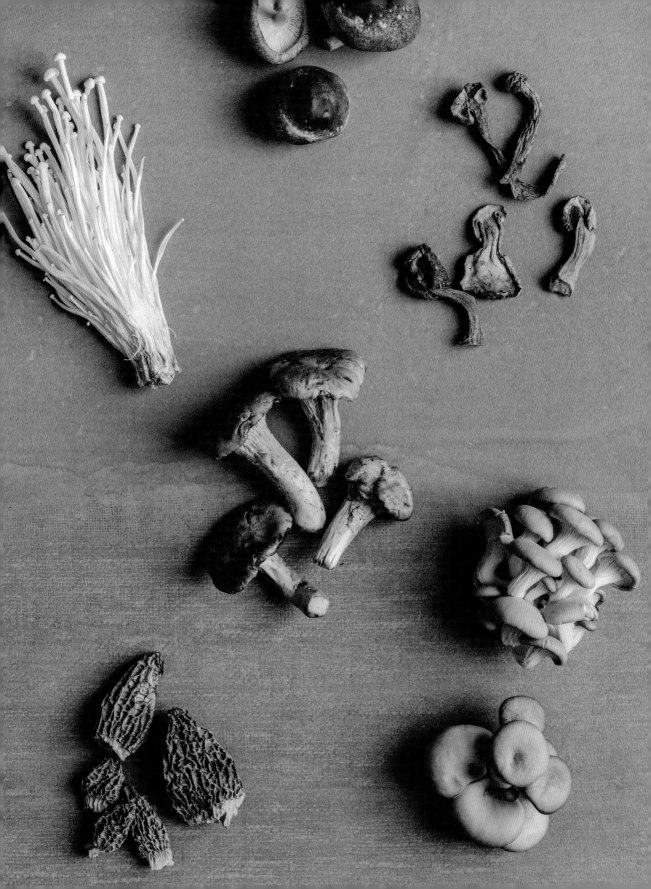

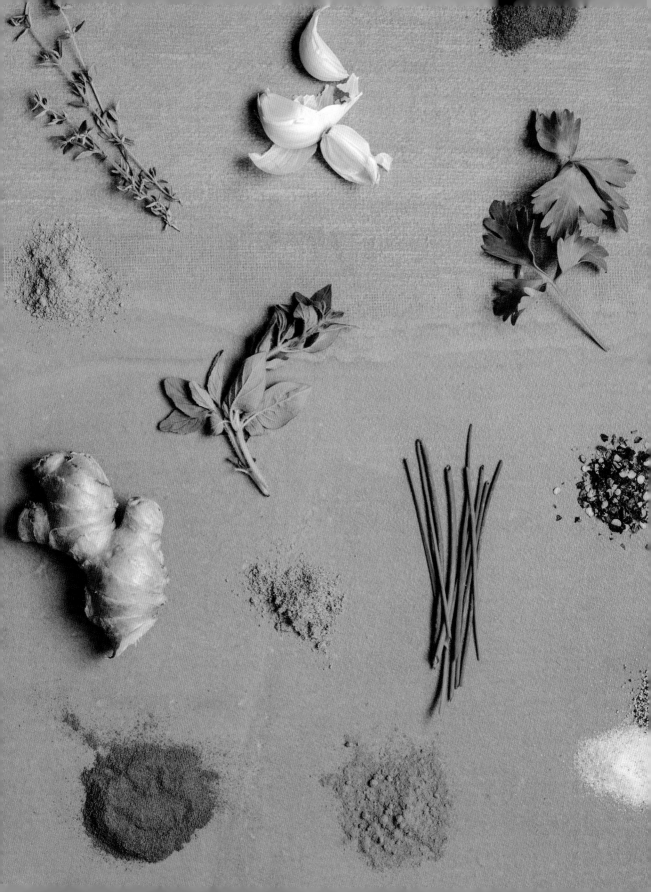

whole spices in bulk and grind them yourself rather than buying small jars of ground spices for ideal flavor and freshness.

STORAGE. Store all dried spices and herbs in airtight jars in a cool, dry pantry. They should stay fresh for about two years. Ground spices typically have a shorter shelf life of six to twelve months. Avoid storing dried herbs and spices above your stove, microwave, refrigerator, or other appliances to avoid unnecessary heat and moisture. Also, I advise against storing bulk dried herbs and spices in the freezer to avoid condensation, which will shorten the lifespan and minimize the flavor.

PREPARATION/COOKING. Remember this formula: 1 tablespoon fresh herbs = 1 teaspoon dried herbs. Crush dried herbs between your fingers before adding them to foods for maximum flavor. Follow your recipe or start adding herbs and spices to your dish in ¼- or ½-teaspoon measurements and increase until you reach your desired taste. To maximize flavor, add dried whole spices early in the cooking process and fresh herbs toward the end. If you're using ground spices, consider adding them to the cooking oil in a sauté pan and heating on low to medium heat for about 30 seconds before adding the other ingredients. The fat-soluble flavor compounds will "bloom" in the heated oil, increasing the overall flavor and aroma of the spices in your dish.

Canned, Jarred, and Nonperishable
Bone broth, canned tuna, canned beans, unsweetened coconut cream/full-fat coconut milk, poultry and/or vegetable stock, soy milk, canned tomatoes (whole and diced), tomato sauce, tomato paste

These are convenient, nonperishable ingredients that I recommend having on hand to supplement your fresh and frozen pantry items. Homemade versions of these are a fantastic choice, but when life doesn't allow for that, commercial versions may just save the day! Consider the same food-as-medicine guidelines, including the Dirty Dozen/Clean Fifteen and sustainability, when purchasing these foods. Also, consider buying various brands and comparing them to find the one you prefer.

Whenever possible, prioritize BPA-free cans to avoid plastic linings that have been shown to leach harmful toxins into food. Be sure to read the labels on these products, since many of them often include unnecessary and questionable ingredients. Buy "low sodium" or "no salt added" options whenever possible, and add your own seasonings after opening.

Store unopened canned, jarred, and nonperishable items in a cool, dry pantry. They will keep for years, even decades. Once they're opened, cover and store them in your refrigerator for the allotted amount of time noted on the jar or bottle by the manufacturing company. When in doubt, look closely and do a smell check. Food within a safe window of time should, but does not always, appear as expected and have a minimal, pleasant, and subtle smell. There should be no slime or mold, and it should not smell overly pungent, sharp, or rancid.

PREPARATION/COOKING. Preparation and cooking information varies greatly for each of these ingredients, depending on the brand, recipe, and specific culinary uses.

Condiments

Fish sauce, gochujang paste (Korean red chili paste), Dijon mustard, whole grain mustard, nutritional yeast, sea salt (fine, coarse)

These ingredients are some of my favorite flavor makers! They are the perfect addition for marinades, dressings, sauces, and more. They can elevate your food, highlight specific ingredients, and create general flavor bombs. Experiment with each one before adding it to your food. Taste a little on a spoon or dip your clean finger into the jar to better understand the flavor profile, especially of an ingredient you've never tried before.

When considering salt, I recommend choosing unrefined sea salt due to the increased mineral content and its lack of exposure to chemicals and potentially harmful manufacturing processes. Unrefined sea salt often contains colored flecks or bits and pieces of actual trace minerals.

STORAGE. There are various recommendations for storing these ingredients. Look on the packaging for each one for more information and for the "Best By" date for optimal freshness and food safety.

PREPARATION/COOKING. Add small amounts of these ingredients to your food at first and continue to taste, adding more as needed as you cook. Remember, you can always add more, but you can't reverse what's already been done! With salt, consider using fine sea salt for seasoning your food along the way and the coarse or flaked variety as a finishing salt. Finishing salt is salt that you sprinkle on your food after it's been prepared or cooked, right

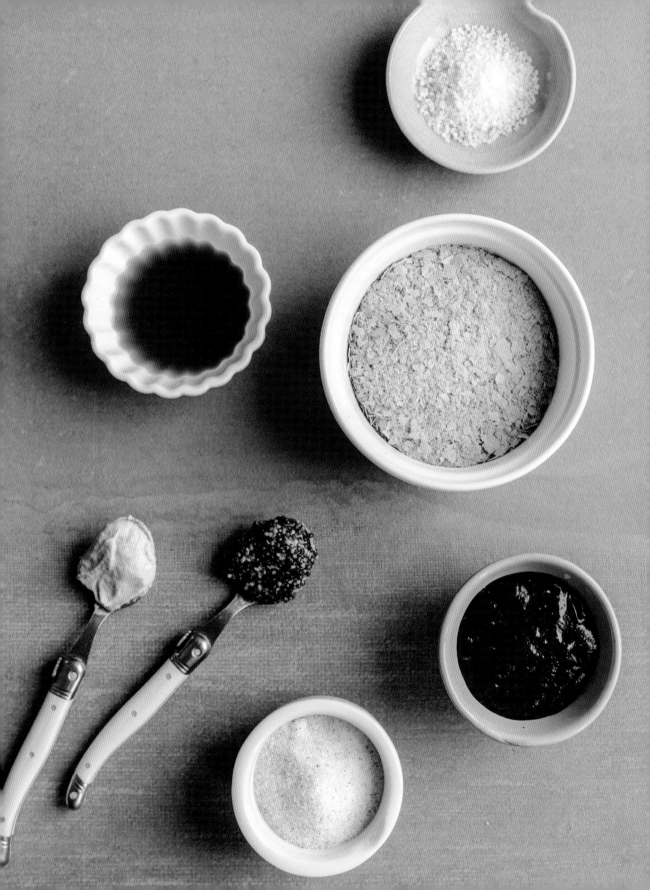

before you serve it. Typically, finishing salt is large grained, and you can see it sitting on top of the finished dish, like with Cashew Butter Stuffed Dates with Dark Chocolate and Sea Salt (page 209).

Vinegars

Apple cider vinegar, balsamic vinegar, sherry vinegar, red/white wine vinegar, rice vinegar

Vinegar adds depth of flavor, acid, and brightness to any dish. It's a fantastic addition to salad dressings, marinades, pickles, sautéed vegetables, soups, and so much more. Choose naturally fermented, unfiltered, and unpasteurized vinegars whenever possible to preserve the highest nutrient content. Unfiltered unpasteurized vinegars also deliver friendly bacteria or probiotics and some antioxidants for an extra nutritional boost, whereas many commercially manufactured vinegars do not or have only very small amounts. Some vinegars, like authentically aged balsamic, are still made and preserved as traditional "slow" ferments, taking months or even years to ferment, which improves the flavor and nutritional value. In either form, read labels and make sure your vinegar doesn't contain any unnecessary ingredients like artificial coloring or preservatives.

STORAGE. You can store most vinegars, unopened or opened, in a dry, cool pantry for multiple years. Just note, they will slowly lose their potency and flavor over time.

PREPARATION/COOKING. Vinegar can be heated and cooked (although some chefs think it's a waste of a precious substance) or left raw. In my opinion, vinegar really shines when kept fresh as a last-minute addition or drizzle.

Baking

Aluminum-free baking powder, arrowroot, baking soda, unsweetened cacao (nibs, powder), dark chocolate (bar, chips), dry yeast, vanilla extract, whole wheat and other whole grain flours

This is an area of your pantry where you need to keep a watchful eye. Baking ingredients are often overly processed and laden with added and unnecessary ingredients such as aluminum (yikes!) and chemical anticaking agents. Look for minimally processed ingredients whenever possible.

STORAGE. You can store most of your baking ingredients in a cool, dry pantry in airtight containers or sealed bags. Shelf life will vary greatly between products. Whole grain flours, such as whole wheat flour, for example, will last in a cool dry pantry for one to three months or in your refrigerator or freezer for up to six months. You want to keep dry yeast in the refrigerator as well.

PREPARATION/COOKING. Don't be afraid of baking or the ingredients used in baking. Making muffins, quick breads, cakes, and crisps can be a great way to add wholesome ingredients to your diet. There are endless baking recipes out there that you can experiment with using a variety of healthy ingredients—surely there's one for you! Try my recipes for Mini Whole Wheat Apple Galettes with Salted Honey (page 183) or Carrot Cake Cupcakes with Vanilla Tofu Frosting (page 137).

Sweeteners

Unsweetened applesauce, unrefined organic cane sugar, dates, date sugar, unfiltered unpasteurized honey, maple syrup, maple sugar, unsulphured blackstrap molasses

Choose unrefined sweeteners for all of your sweetening needs whenever possible. This means the sweetener has been processed less and may even still contain some nutrients (true!). Consider blackstrap molasses, for example. It's one of the first extractions from sugarcane and includes notable amounts of iron, manganese, magnesium, potassium, and copper. Make sure you choose unsulphured molasses to minimize the environmental impact of sugar cane and molasses production and to avoid the addition of sulfur dioxide, a potentially harmful additive used to extend the shelf life.

However, most sweeteners have to go through some type of processing, so pay attention to the form of the sweetener you buy and always read the label. It may benefit you to read more about specific brands, their processing techniques, and sustainability. My preferred go-to sweetener is unpasteurized or "raw" honey fresh from the hive with only mild processing to remove any natural debris and/or bee parts.

STORAGE. Store your sweeteners in a cool, dry pantry in airtight containers that are free from moisture. Many well-kept sweeteners will last for two to three years or indefinitely, like honey.

PREPARATION/COOKING. There are a variety of ways to use each sweetener. Applesauce can be added to baked goods that need extra moisture and sweetness like cake. Dates can be blended into smoothies, or date sugar can be added to cookies. You can use sweeteners in both uncooked prepared foods or baked and cooked dishes. A touch of sweetness can balance a dish, so consider adding a splash or sprinkle to salad dressings, soups, or sauces for a more rounded flavor.

Shopping

Once you have a better idea of what you want to include in your pantry, it's time to go shopping. This is always my favorite part. Many people loathe grocery shopping, but I challenge you to find a way to make it fun—or at least interesting. I've included many tips here to help expedite this process, keep you focused, sort through all the options, and save you money. Whether you shop at a farmer's market, cooperative, or grocery store, use these tips as a guide. I've also included a couple of suggestions for making more conscious choices in consideration of the environment.

- Review your pantry, fridge, and freezer before making a shopping list.

- Plan ahead or create a meal plan.

- Write a shopping list to keep yourself organized and save time and money.

- Eat a snack or meal before you go shopping so you're more likely to stick to your list and avoid unnecessary "impulse" purchases.

- Take your time.

- Prioritize seasonal and local whole foods whenever possible.

- Fill your cart or basket with naturally colorful foods—rainbow foods!

- Fresh, frozen, and canned foods are all OK choices.

- When considering meat or seafood, consider buying the same product from the freezer section rather than at the counter, where prices may be higher and the shelf life shorter.

- Read labels and look for minimally processed foods with few ingredients.

- Take note of your preferred brands, farmers, and so on to make shopping easier and faster next time.

- Experiment with new ingredients and spices by buying small amounts in the bulk section before committing to larger packaged quantities.

- Only buy what you want—ask your produce manager or butcher to portion food that's priced by weight, such as meat and produce. (Do you need only half of a head of cabbage?)

- Ask your butcher to grind meat fresh for you or provide you with bones for homemade bone broth.

- Ask the department manager to stock your favorite brand or ingredient if the store doesn't already do so.

- Save money (usually) by buying directly from the farmer or look for the grocery store's brand if they have one.

- Consider product placement and how this may affect pricing. Some food manufacturers actually pay supermarkets more for premium shelf space that's typically central and eye-level to increase profits.

- Review unit prices for better deals and look for sales.

- Only buy what you need—you can always come back for more.

- Bring your own reusable jars/containers for bulk items (this saves you a step at home too!), just make sure to use the tare function on a digital scale before adding your bulk goods so that you're not unnecessarily paying for the weight of your container.

- Use reusable cloth produce bags and avoid using plastic bags whenever possible.

- Bring reusable grocery bags, or recycle your paper bags.

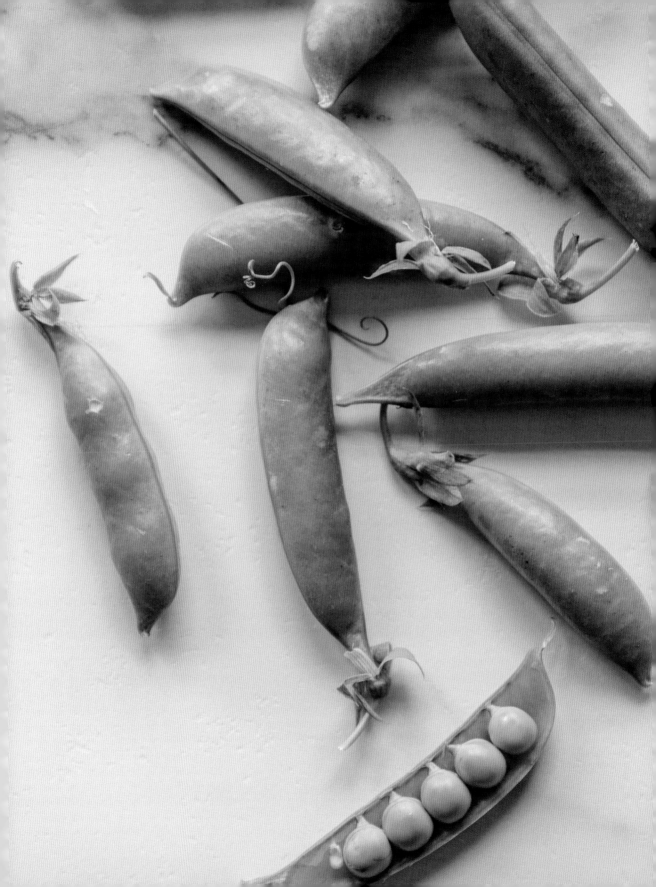

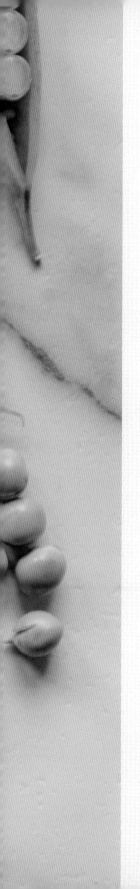

PART TWO

RECIPES

5

RECIPES FOR ALL SEASONS

These are foundational recipes found in a well-rounded whole foods kitchen and are staples in my household. They hold their own year-round and can flex and bend as the seasons come and go. Milk, yogurt, beans, nut butter—all virtuous foods that make eating a whole foods diet that much easier (and tastier!). I recommend having most or all of these recipes readily available at a moment's notice. You can prepare them in batches and stock the surplus in your refrigerator or pantry for later use—a scoop of beans here, a dollop of yogurt there. As the seasons change, you can make slight adjustments or adaptations to celebrate and highlight the current season. Add strawberries to the almond milk in the late spring or quick pickle some beets in the autumn.

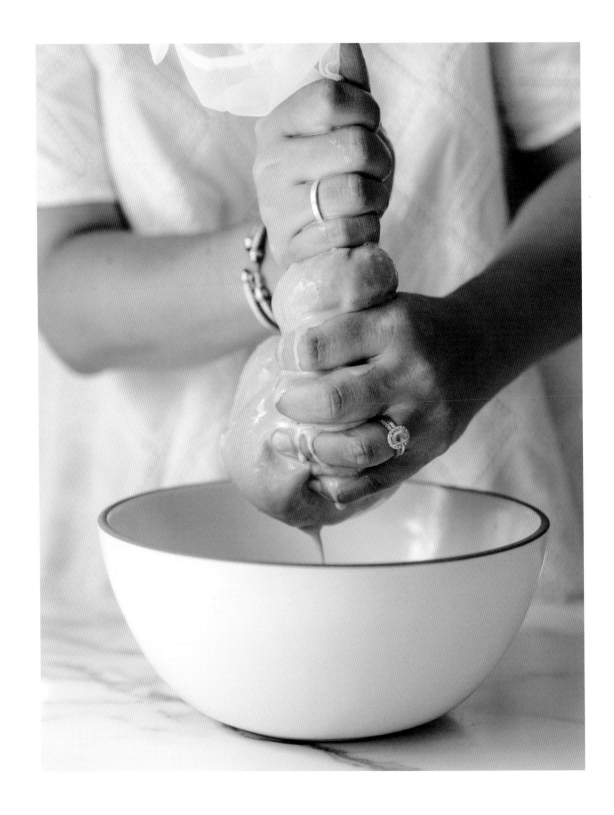

Almond Milk
(and Strawberry Almond Milk)

This almond milk is creamier and tastier than any version you can find at your local grocery store, *and* it only has five ingredients. Not only is it nutrient dense and full of healthy fats and protein, but it's also a blank canvas for any flavor profile. Keep it plain or add seasonal berries, like I do here, for a fruity version or add unsweetened cocoa powder to make decadent chocolate almond milk.

You'll need a high-powered blender to blend the ingredients, as well as a cotton nut milk bag, fine cheesecloth, or a thin dish towel to strain them. MAKES 6 CUPS

DF | GF | V | Ve | RT

2 cups raw almonds

5 cups water

2 tablespoons maple syrup

1 teaspoon vanilla extract

¼ teaspoon sea salt

1 pound fresh or frozen strawberries, hulled (optional)

Place your almonds in a large glass bowl and cover with room-temperature water. Soak overnight or for at least 8 hours until plump and hydrated (you should have about 3 cups once they're hydrated).

Drain and rinse the soaked almonds and place with all other ingredients in a blender. Add optional flavor variations, such as strawberries, now. You may need to make your almond milk in batches if you have a small blender. Blend on high for 2 minutes or until thoroughly blended. The longer you blend your ingredients, the more nutrients you'll extract from the almonds.

Place a cotton nut milk bag, double layer of fine cheesecloth, or thin dish towel over a large bowl; pour the almond milk mixture into it and gently squeeze the contents, separating the milk from the pulp. This may require two or three batches to avoid overflow. Once you're done, set the pulp aside and pour the almond milk into two separate quart jars or glass containers with lids; store in the refrigerator. Fresh almond milk will keep for 3 to 5 days. Shake well before serving.

> Save your nut milk pulp and dehydrate it in the oven with herbs and salt to make gluten-free "breadcrumbs" for roasted veggies or pasta, or make a natural body scrub by adding the pulp to coarse sea salt, coconut oil, and a few drops of your favorite essential oil(s).

Bone Broth (Chicken)

Chicken soup or broth may truly be the best thing to cure the common cold. Research shows that it contains anti-inflammatory properties that slow down or even stop cold symptoms. Bone broth is also rich in amino acids and electrolytes, making it a fantastic sports recovery drink for those who need an extra boost or for mamas during labor and delivery and in their early postpartum days. It's OK to mix different animal bones (chicken, cow, and so on) to make your bone broth, but keep in mind that the benefits of bone broth have only been shown effective with chicken bones. MAKES ABOUT 4 QUARTS (SERVING SIZE WILL VARY)

DF | GF | RT

1 whole previously cooked chicken carcass or any other bones, meat removed

Water

1 tablespoon apple cider vinegar

3 celery stalks, roughly chopped

2 large carrots, roughly chopped

1 medium white or yellow onion (peel on OK), roughly chopped

4 whole garlic cloves (peel on OK)

1 lemon, quartered

Your favorite fresh herbs (thyme, parsley, rosemary, bay leaves)

Sea salt and ground black pepper to taste

Preheat oven to 450°F. Place the chicken carcass or other types of bones on a baking sheet and roast until the bones have browned, about 30 to 40 minutes, depending on the size and amount of bones. Consider using bones that are naturally high in collagen, such as knuckles, feet, and marrow bones.

Place the roasted bones in a slow cooker or Dutch oven and cover completely with water and vinegar; let sit for 1 hour (no heat). This allows time for the vinegar to leach minerals from the bones. After 1 hour, add celery, carrots, onion, garlic, lemon, and fresh herbs, with additional water if needed to keep the contents covered.

Turn your slow cooker on high or your stove on high heat and bring the broth to a boil. Skim off any foam that accumulates on the surface. Reduce heat to low, cover, and let simmer for at least 24 hours. For better flavor and a more potent, mineral-rich broth, let simmer for 48 hours. Check your broth intermittently to skim off foam and add more water if necessary.

After 24 to 48 hours, turn your slow cooker off or remove your Dutch oven from the heat and let it cool slightly before handling. Using a large colander or fine mesh strainer, carefully strain your broth into a large bowl, discarding the bones and all other ingredients. Season the broth to your liking with salt and pepper before pouring into individual jars or containers. Let the broth cool completely before adding lids and storing in your refrigerator for 7 to 10 days or in your freezer, leaving 1 to 2 inches of headspace, for up to one year.

> Use well-sourced, high-quality bones for the best broth. Ask your local butcher or farmer for bones and/or save your bones from recipes like Whole Roasted Chicken with Maple Root Vegetables on page 201).

Ghee

Ghee is butter that's been heated and strained to remove the milk solids or proteins (casein and whey). Those with a dairy intolerance can often tolerate ghee since the problematic proteins have been taken out, leaving only the butter fat. By removing the milk solids, you are also increasing the smoke point of the butter, providing an end product with more diverse applications like high-heat frying and roasting. MAKES 12 OUNCES

GF | V

1 pound unsalted butter

Melt the butter in a saucepan over low to medium heat. Once it is completely melted, the butter will begin to separate into three distinct layers—milk solids on the bottom and top and butter fat or oil in the middle. Using a large spoon, gently skim and remove the foaming milk solids on the surface and discard. You should have two layers left.

At this point, don't stir and disrupt the two layers. Allow them to stay separate while continuing to simmer, skimming any stray solids on the top. Eventually, the top translucent oil layer will turn a golden-brown color. Don't rush this step: this is what imparts that delicious, toasty ghee flavor. Continue simmering the butter oil until you reach your desired flavor and color (I prefer 6 to 8 minutes).

Turn off the heat, and prepare a small mesh strainer and a 16-ounce glass jar with a lid. Line your strainer with fine cheesecloth and place over your jar. Carefully and slowly pour the golden butter oil through the cheesecloth and strainer into the jar, leaving any milk solids in the pan. Discard the remaining solids. What you're left with is liquid ghee. It will solidify at room temperature where you can keep it for 2 to 3 months, or you can store it in the refrigerator for up to 1 year.

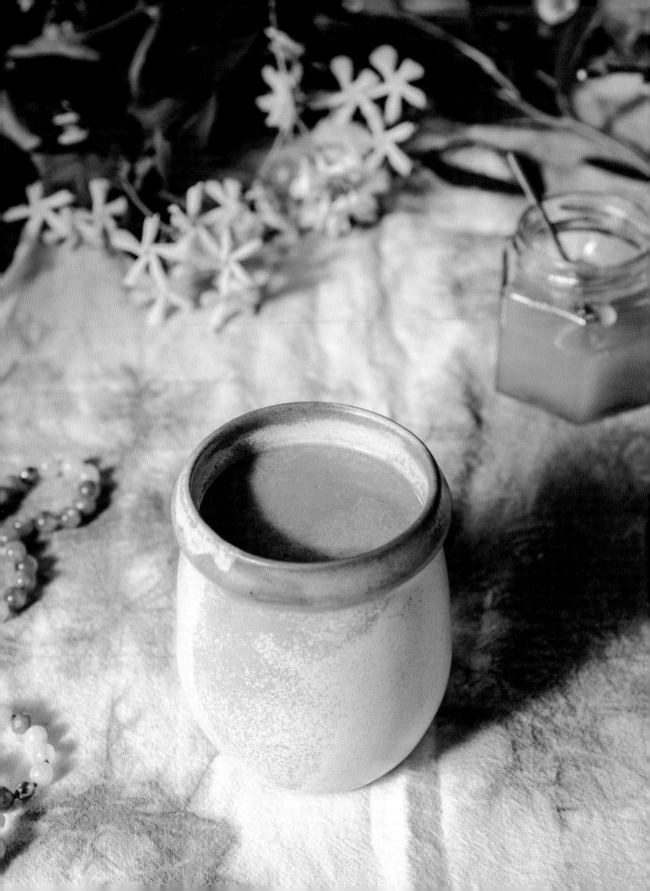

Golden Turmeric Paste

Worth its weight in gold! This stuff is a fantastic addition to your morning latte, favorite soup, curry, or fried rice. Turmeric contains a bioactive compound called curcumin, which is best known for its powerful anti-inflammatory and antioxidant benefits. Black pepper aids in the absorption of curcumin, so always make sure to include some in recipes calling for turmeric.

MAKES 8 OUNCES

DF | GF | V | Ve

⅓ cup ground turmeric

1½ teaspoons ground ginger

1 teaspoon ground cardamom

½ teaspoon ground cinnamon

¼ teaspoon ground black pepper

¾ cup water

¼ cup coconut oil

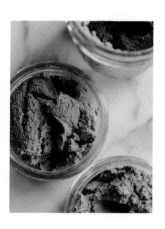

In a small bowl, whisk together the turmeric, ginger, cardamom, cinnamon, and pepper. Add the water to a small saucepan on low to medium heat, and whisk in the turmeric mixture until smooth. Continue to whisk while heating the mixture for 3 to 4 minutes or until it reduces slightly. Remove from the heat and whisk in the coconut oil until it's fully melted and incorporated, about 1 minute. Your paste should be thick but smooth and pourable at this point. Pour the mixture into an 8-ounce glass jar and let it cool, uncovered, to room temperature. Once cool, add the lid and refrigerate for up to one month. Let paste come to room temperature before using.

For **golden milk**, add 1 to 2 teaspoons of Golden Turmeric Paste to 1 cup of your preferred milk in a small saucepan and heat on low to medium heat. Whisk until they are incorporated, and heat to the desired temperature. Add your sweetener of choice if desired. Pour into a mug and enjoy.

For **curry**, add 2 tablespoons of Golden Turmeric Paste after you sauté your protein and vegetables, just before adding your coconut milk and any other liquids. The turmeric paste will replace the curry paste in other recipes.

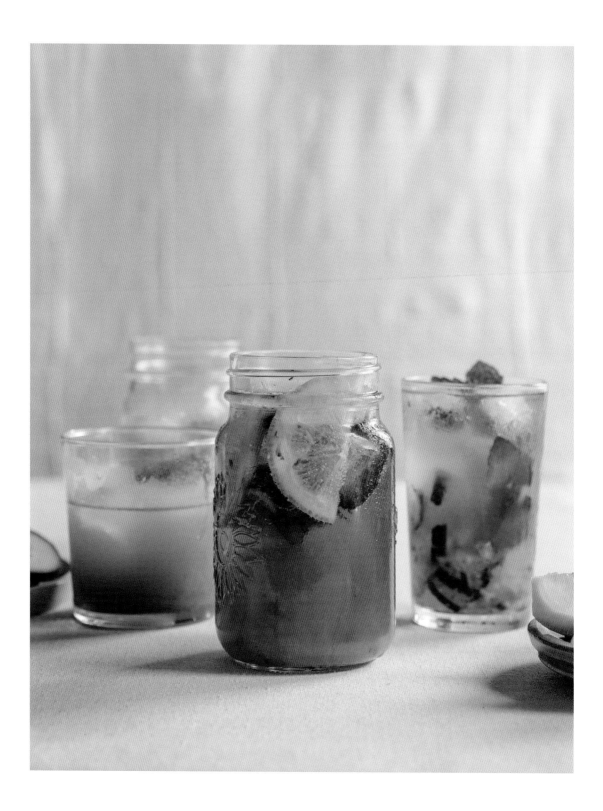

Infused Water

Staying hydrated doesn't have to be boring or translate to drinking only ice water or sugary sports drinks in large quantities. Infused water is a fantastic way to help you meet your daily fluid needs. Get creative and have fun with different concoctions, including fruit and vegetable infusions and recipes that use sparkling water (yes, sparkling water counts!).

SERVES 2 (PER RECIPE)

DF | GF | V | Ve

Ice

4 strawberries, hulled and sliced

2 cups lightly sweetened lemonade

4 cups plain sparkling water

1 lemon, thinly sliced crosswise (garnish)

Sparkling Strawberry Lemonade

Fill two glasses with ice and set aside. In a metal shaker, muddle the strawberries with a small scoop of ice. Add the lemonade and cover tightly with the lid. Shake vigorously for 30 seconds. Divide the contents into the glasses with ice and top each with equal amounts of sparkling water. Garnish each with a lemon slice.

Ice

1½ cups green juice

1½ cups still water or plain or orange/tangerine flavored sparkling water

½ lime, cut into wedges

Green Juice Infusion

Fill two glasses with ice. Divide the green juice evenly between the glasses and finish with still or sparkling water. Top off each glass with a squeeze of lime.

Ice

12 mint leaves, plus more for garnish

½ cucumber, sliced crosswise into ¼-inch-thick pieces

Juice of 1 lime

1 cup coconut water

2 tablespoons maple syrup (optional)

1½ cups plain or lime-flavored sparkling water

Coconut "Faux-Jito"

Fill two glasses with ice and set aside. In a large metal shaker, muddle the mint and 4 slices of cucumber with a small scoop of ice. Add the lime juice, coconut water, and optional sweetener, and cover tightly with the lid. Shake vigorously for 30 seconds. Divide the contents between the glasses of ice and top with sparkling water. Garnish with whole mint leaves and additional slices of cucumber.

Lacto-Fermented Vegetables: Two Ways

Besides being incredibly addicting, these lacto-fermented vegetables are loaded with healthy bacteria, also known as probiotics, which are extremely beneficial to your health. Originally used as a method of food preservation, fermentation has become a health food staple, delivering powerful lactobacilli (bacteria) directly to your kitchen and, thus, to your body.

MAKES 1 QUART-SIZE JAR (PER RECIPE)

DF | GF | V | Ve | RT

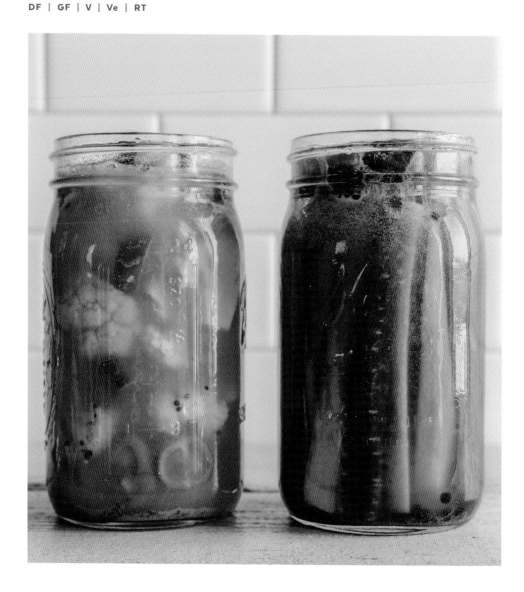

Curried Cauliflower

½ head cauliflower, cut into florets

5 small sweet red peppers, sliced crosswise

3 cloves garlic, smashed

2⅓ cups water

5 teaspoons sea salt

1 teaspoon ground turmeric

1 teaspoon black or brown mustard seeds

½ teaspoon ground coriander

½ teaspoon cumin

½ teaspoon red chili flakes

1 cabbage leaf, cut into a circle slightly larger than the size of the jar opening

Garlic Pepper Carrots

10 large rainbow carrots, washed and peeled, ends removed, halved lengthwise, cut into 6-inch spears or sticks

2 garlic cloves, smashed

1⅔ cups water

5 teaspoons sea salt

1 teaspoon black peppercorns

1 cabbage leaf, cut into a circle slightly larger than the size of the jar opening

Choose one recipe or make both simultaneously.

Wash and thoroughly dry a wide-mouth 1-quart glass jar with lid and set aside. In a medium-size bowl, mix together the vegetables and garlic, and pack them into the jar, leaving about ½ inch of headspace on top; add more vegetables as needed. Using the same bowl, make the brine. Add the water, salt, and spices, and mix together using a fork or small whisk. It's OK if some spices don't fully dissolve and settle on the bottom.

Pour the brine over the vegetables, filling the jar to the brim. Place the cabbage leaf inside the jar, on top of the vegetables, to act as a plug to ensure that all of the vegetables are fully immersed in the brine. Some of the brine should spill over and cover the cabbage leaf, creating an anaerobic environment for the fermentation to do its magic. Do not leave any vegetables exposed (other than the cabbage leaf if necessary).

Create an airtight seal on the jar with the lid and store at room temperature out of direct sunlight for 5 to 10 days, or until the vegetables reach your desired flavor. Start to "burp" the jar on day 2 by opening it and releasing the built-up air pressure created from the fermentation process. After burping, quickly reseal the jar and continue to ferment. Burp the jar at least once a day from then on. It's OK if some liquid escapes when you do this. Store the jar on a kitchen towel if necessary. Alternatively, you can use a designated fermentation lid fitted to your jar with a one-way air vent that releases oxygen throughout the day and does away with the need for burping. You can easily find these lids online or at specialty grocery stores.

The best way to tell if the vegetables are ready is to try one! The longer you ferment them, the tangier they will become (I typically prefer a 9- to 10-day ferment). If you're storing and fermenting in a warm room, consider a shorter fermentation time closer to 5 to 6 days. Once you reach your desired tanginess and flavor, move the jar to the refrigerator, where it will stop fermenting and keep for about 6 months.

> You can read more about the health benefits of fermented and cultured foods on page 45.

Nut and Seed Butter

Homemade nut and seed butters are simple and incredibly satisfying to make. It's also a great way to avoid the unnecessary added sugar found in many commercial versions. Making your own nut butter offers more versatility too—you can use one variety of nut or seed or mix two or more together to create more dynamic flavor combinations like almond and walnut butter or macadamia and cashew butter. You can also add spices like cinnamon and cardamom or sweeten your nut butter with honey or maple syrup. Or add maca or reishi powder for something really nontraditional and fun. The possibilities are endless! However, do keep in mind that recipe variations will likely change the consistency of the nut/seed butter requiring more or less nuts/seeds.

Note that you will need a high-quality food processor to grind the nuts for this recipe.

MAKES ABOUT 2 CUPS

DF | GF | V | Ve

3 cups nuts or seeds (or a combination)

Pinch of sea salt

Preheat oven to 300°F. Spread your favorite nuts and/or seeds in a single, even layer on an unlined baking sheet. Roast for 18 to 20 minutes, or until the nuts/seeds are fragrant and lightly toasted. Smaller nuts and seeds may take less time. Remove from the oven and set aside to cool.

When they are cool enough to handle, add the nuts/seeds and salt (and any other spices or sweeteners) to a food processor with a metal chopping, or S, blade. Blend on high for 4 to 5 minutes for smaller or softer nuts/seeds like cashews and walnuts or 10 to 12 minutes for larger or heartier nuts/seeds like almonds and pistachios. Stop the food processor intermittently to scrape down the sides with a rubber spatula. Continue to process until the butter is smooth and creamy. Be patient. The butter will go through various stages before turning into the creamy richness you're used to.

Scrape the finished butter into a pint-size glass jar with a wide mouth and seal with a lid. Eat it by the spoonful, with apple slices, or use it in your favorite recipes like the Flourless Chocolate Almond Butter Brownies (page 161) or Cashew Butter Stuffed Dates with Dark Chocolate and Sea Salt (page 209). Store at room temperature for up to 3 months.

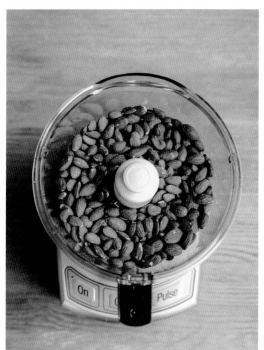

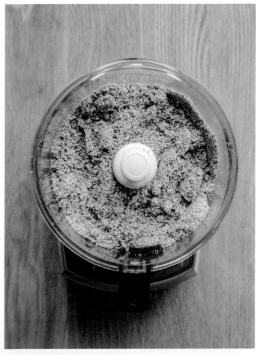

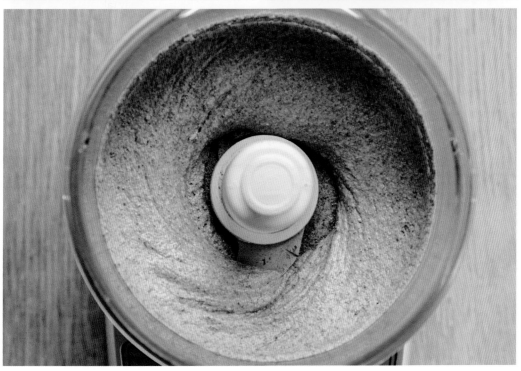

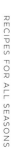

Plain Whole Milk Yogurt

Homemade yogurt is full of healthy bacteria, aka probiotics. It's better tasting than store-bought varieties and better for you since it contains only two ingredients and no added sugar. Once you've made the yogurt, feel free to mix in your favorite flavorings or toppings to make it your own. Some of my favorite variations include mixing in puréed strawberries or mangoes or keeping it simple and adding granola and a swirl of maple syrup. MAKES 4 CUPS

GF | V | RT

4 cups whole milk (cow's, goat's, or sheep's milk)

5 grams yogurt starter culture (or recommended amount per manufacturer, see note)

Many grocery stores carry yogurt starters in the refrigerated section near the commercial yogurt. You can easily order starters online as well. Make sure your yogurt starter is designed for the type of milk you're using (that is, dairy or vegan). Refer to the packaging for the manufacturer's instructions.

Bring the milk to a boil in a small saucepan on high heat, stirring regularly with a wooden spoon to avoid burning the bottom. Once it is boiling, remove from the heat. Using a food thermometer, let the milk cool to 75°F to 80°F. To speed up the cooling process, you can place your hot saucepan in a sink filled with cold or ice water.

Pour about ½ cup cooled milk into a small bowl and add the powdered yogurt culture. Mix well with a small whisk or fork until the starter is fully dissolved. Pour the cultured milk back into the saucepan and mix well with the rest of the milk. Pour all of the cultured milk into a 1-quart glass jar with a wide mouth and seal with an airtight lid.

Switch on the light in the oven but keep the heat off. Place the jar in the oven as close to the light as possible. Feel free to use a yogurt machine or other heat-controlled electric appliance instead if you already have one (follow the appliance instructions), but it's not necessary. Your oven light is a sufficient heat source. Incubate for 18 to 20 hours, or until the yogurt becomes firm and easily pulls away from the side of the jar. Check your yogurt intermittently throughout this process. The longer you incubate the yogurt, the firmer and tangier or more sour it will become. If you let the yogurt incubate for too long (typically over 24 hours), it can curdle and become lumpy. Although, this can be fixed easily by straining it through a fine mesh strainer or cheesecloth to remove any solids.

Check out the recipe for Cultured Key Lime Cashew Yogurt on page 143 for an alternative vegan yogurt-making method.

Once you've reached your desired taste and texture, remove from the oven and refrigerate for 8 hours or overnight to stop incubation and cool the yogurt. Scoop out your desired serving size and serve cold with your favorite additions or toppings. Try some on top of the Beef and Beet Borscht with Fresh Beet Greens (page 181) or on top of the Spicy Three Bean Chili (page 197).

When you're ready to make a new batch, reserve ½ cup of yogurt from the current batch and use this as your starter for the new batch (instead of the manufactured yogurt starter). Do this by dissolving ½ cup of reserved yogurt into ½ cup cooled milk from the new batch in a small bowl and then add it back into the total mixture before incubating. You can "recycle" or reculture your yogurt like this, in theory, indefinitely. However, keep in mind that the reserved yogurt starter needs to be reused and reincubated fairly promptly or the cultures will die.

Quick Vinegar Pickles (Carrots)

These quick pickles are a great way to add more flavor and texture to your meals. Try some on a green salad or on fish tacos for an additional zip. Remember, these do not contain probiotics like their fermented friends, but they sure are good! Read more about pickling versus fermentation on page 46. MAKES 1 QUART-SIZE JAR (PER RECIPE)

DF | GF | V | Ve | RT

1 pound large carrots

1 cup water

1 cup apple cider vinegar

2 tablespoons maple syrup

1 tablespoon yellow mustard seeds

2 teaspoons whole allspice berries

2 teaspoons black peppercorns

½ teaspoon ground coriander

1 teaspoon sea salt

Slice your carrots on a diagonal or bias cut into ⅛-inch "coins" (I like to use a mandoline). This will yield about 3 cups of carrots. Add them to a 1-quart glass jar with a wide mouth and lid; set aside.

In a small saucepan on medium to high heat, combine water, vinegar, maple syrup, and all of the spices, including the salt; bring to a gentle boil. As soon as the liquid boils, remove from the heat and pour the brine into the jar with the carrots. (It should completely cover the carrots. If not, add a splash of hot water to top it off.) Let the carrots and brine cool to room temperature before adding the lid. Give the jar a couple of shakes to evenly distribute the spices and then place in the refrigerator. Cool thoroughly before enjoying. Store in the refrigerator for up to 6 months.

> You can use carrots sticks instead of "coins" or another vegetable such as sliced red onion, cauliflower florets, rainbow chard stems, whole cherry tomatoes, or asparagus spears.

Cooking Beans and Legumes

Preparing dried beans and legumes from scratch is so worth the extra time. Compared to canned beans, the flavor and texture of home-cooked beans is by far superior. Use the table below as a helpful guide when cooking beans and legumes. Remember to wash and rinse your beans thoroughly before cooking them to remove any debris. Also, depending on the age of the beans, your cooking time may need to be adjusted—older beans can take hours to cook.

Beans (1 cup dry)	Water or Broth (cups)	Cook Time (without soaking)	Yield (cups)
Adzuki (aduki)	4	45-55 minutes	3
Black	4	1-1½ hours	2-2½
Black-eyed peas	3	1 hour	2
Cannellini	3	45 minutes	2½
Chickpeas	4	1-3 hours	2
Corona	4	1½-2 hours	3
Great Northern	3½	1½ hours	2½-3
Kidney beans	3	1 hour	2-2½
Lentils, brown	2¼	20-25 minutes	2-2½
Lentils, green	2	20-25 minutes	2
Lentils, red	3	15-20 minutes	2-2½
Mung	2½	1 hour	2
Navy	3	45-60 minutes	2½-3
Pinto	3	1-1½ hours	2½-3
Soy	4	3-4 hours	3

Soaking

Beans and legumes naturally contain a type of carbohydrate called oligosaccharides that can cause gas (the musical fruit!). Studies show that soaking dried beans for at least 12 hours or overnight before cooking may reduce some of the gas-producing properties. If you're unable to soak your dried beans first, consider adding a small piece of kombu seaweed (found at most Asian markets and natural-food stores) during cooking to neutralize the difficult-to-digest compounds. Kombu also lends a nice salty flavor and improves the overall texture of the beans. Brining beans in a salt solution overnight can also create a more tender, smoother consistency, so there's another benefit of overnight soaking.

Cooking on the Stovetop

This is the conventional way to cook beans and legumes. Whether you soaked your beans first or not, you will start the same way. Depending on the amount of beans you're cooking, add them to a medium or large saucepan with a lid or a Dutch oven. Reference the chart and add as much water or broth as necessary (make sure your beans are covered by at least 1 inch of liquid). You may need more liquid if you are using soaked beans, since they will typically double or even triple in their original size.

Bring the liquid/bean mixture to a boil on high heat. Once boiling, reduce the heat to low and simmer—you know you're at the right temperature when you can barely see anything happening in the pan. Cover your saucepan with a lid and let the beans simmer for the allotted time per the chart. If using soaked beans, you can expect the cooking time to be shorter. Check for doneness—the beans should be tender but not mushy and should hold their shape. Continue to cook if necessary, adding more liquid to keep the beans covered until done. Tip: Check at least five different beans or a small spoonful, as some beans will cook faster or slower than the others depending on their age.

Cooking with a Pressure Cooker

Pressure cooking dried beans and legumes can save you a significant amount of time. In general, you will need to add more water to the beans than with the stovetop method. Follow the manufacturer's instructions for specific cooking times since each pressure cooker varies slightly. Most beans and legumes will cook in a pressure cooker in 25 to 40 minutes.

Cooking Whole Grains

Cooking whole grains is fairly straightforward, although the cooking times vary slightly between grains. The following table can be a really helpful tool until you find your own confidence and rhythm in preparing them. Before cooking, remember to wash and rinse your grains thoroughly until the water runs clear to eliminate dirt and excess starch.

Grain (1 cup dry)	Water or Broth (cups)	Cook Time (without soaking)	Yield (cups)
Amaranth	2	25 minutes	3½
Barley	3	45–60 minutes	3½
Buckwheat	2	20 minutes	4
Jasmine Rice	1½	20 minutes	3½–4
Millet	2½	20 minutes	4
Oats, rolled	2	10 minutes	1½
Oats, steel-cut	3	20–30 minutes	4
Pasta, whole wheat	6	8–12 minutes	Varies
Polenta (corn grits)	4	25–30 minutes	2½
Quinoa	2	12–15 minutes	3
Brown rice, long-grain	1¾	45–50 minutes	3½–4
Brown rice, short-grain	1¾	45–50 minutes	3½–4
Spelt	4	45–60 minutes	3
Teff	3	20 minutes	3
Wheat berries	4	45–60 minutes	3
Wild rice	3	45–55 minutes	3½

Soaking

Soaking any type of whole grain in water for at least 8 hours or overnight before cooking is highly recommended. Rinse and drain before cooking. Soaked grains will not only cook more quickly, but they are also easier to digest since soaking can help to remove naturally occurring phytic acid, which can inhibit absorption and protein digestion.

Cooking on the Stovetop

This is the conventional way to cook grains. Whether you soaked your grains first or not, you will start the same way. Add the grains to a small or medium saucepan with a lid. Reference the chart and add as much water or broth as necessary depending on the type of grain. Soaked grains will require less liquid and cooking time, although the amount of liquid and cooking time of all grains (soaked or unsoaked) varies greatly depending on the age of the grain, the type of grain, and what type of pan you're using to cook. The key is to test the texture along the way using the chart to estimate liquid measurements and cooking times—simply add more liquid if necessary or drain excess liquid if needed.

Bring the liquid/grain mixture to a boil on high heat and then reduce the heat to low to simmer. Cover your pan and let cook for the allotted time per the chart or slightly less for soaked grains. Avoid opening it unnecessarily to peek along the way, as this will release steam which helps the grains cook evenly. Check for doneness by sampling a small spoonful. The grains should be tender but slightly al dente or firm. Alternatively, you can tilt your pan to the side at an angle—there should be little-to-no liquid remaining in the pan. If liquid remains, and the texture is still too firm, put the lid back on and continue to simmer, checking again in 2- to 3-minute increments until done.

Cooking with the Pasta Method

This is an alternative way to cook grains. This is when you add a dry whole grain to a large pot of boiling water and cook until tender, just like you would with pasta. When the grains are tender, you strain them in a colander and voila! This will reduce the cooking time significantly for many types of whole grains.

Batch Cooking: Cook Once, Eat Multiple Times

Batch cooking is when you cook double or triple (or more multiples of) the required portion of whole grains, beans, veggies, and/or almost any other ingredient as well as full meals and store the surplus in airtight containers in the refrigerator; you can also freeze individual serving sizes. Then, at a later time when you're in need of whole grains or a quick meal, and you don't have the time or inclination to cook, you already have nutritious and delicious foods prepared. Just heat and serve.

Batch cooking is something I can't promote enough! It's a tool that I literally recommend to almost every patient and stranger alike (one example is Spicy Sriracha Mung Bean Bowl with Pickled Daikon and Carrots on page 127).

Growing Sprouts

Growing your own edible sprouts or microgreens is one of the easiest and most nutritionally rewarding techniques you can learn. Three of my favorite sprouting seeds are broccoli, buckwheat, and radish seeds. They're flavorful and easy to grow, making them all great starter seeds for your first-time sprouting adventure or favorites to revisit later as a pro. Most sprouts are rich in antioxidants and various other vitamins and minerals. Preliminary research on edible sprouts, specifically broccoli sprouts, shows powerful anticancer properties too.

MAKES ABOUT 4 CUPS

3–4 tablespoons
    sprouting seeds

Water

DAY 1

Place the seeds in a clean 1-quart glass jar with a wide mouth and cover with room temperature or cool water. Cover loosely with cheesecloth and fasten with a rubber band or a metal jar ring (without the lid insert). Alternatively, you can use a sprouting jar screen lid, which you can easily purchase online. Give the seeds and water a delicate swirl and let them sit at room temperature, out of direct sunlight, for at least 8 hours or overnight.

DAY 2

After soaking the seeds, tip the jar upside down and thoroughly drain out the water through the cheesecloth or screen; rinse the seeds with fresh water and drain again. Prop the jar upside down in a small bowl with the cheesecloth or screen on the bottom, creating an angle for any residual water to drain out. Leave in this position for 4 to 6 hours and then repeat this process, rinsing and draining the seeds. Prop your jar upside down once more and leave overnight.

DAYS 3 TO 8

Rinse and drain your seeds twice daily for a total of 3 to 8 days, until your sprouts start to grow and each sprout is more than 1 inch long. Each variety of seed will take a different amount of time to reach this stage. For example, broccoli seeds typically take 5 to 6 days to sprout, buckwheat seeds 6 to 8 days, and radish seeds around 4 to 5 days. Once they're done sprouting, remove the sprouts and place them in a salad spinner or fine mesh colander; rinse once more before drying them thoroughly. Enjoy raw sprouts on salads, sandwiches, or in your favorite grain bowl. Store sprouts in an airtight (dry) container in your refrigerator for up to 3 to 5 days.

6

SPRING

Spring is the time for awakening and new growth—
like little green buds shooting up through the earth.
As the daylight lengthens, our inner fire is stoked and
we rise to the occasion. We slowly make our way out
into the light and find ourselves renewed and ready.

Our appetite is quenched with smaller more frequent meals. Easy-to-digest foods and gentle detoxification are welcome. Rich and fatty foods are slowly
replaced with lighter meals of delicate and bitter
greens, whole grains, plant proteins, and mushrooms.
Rhubarb, asparagus, dandelion, nettles, fiddlehead
ferns, morels—a celebratory bounty to enliven and
stimulate the taste buds.

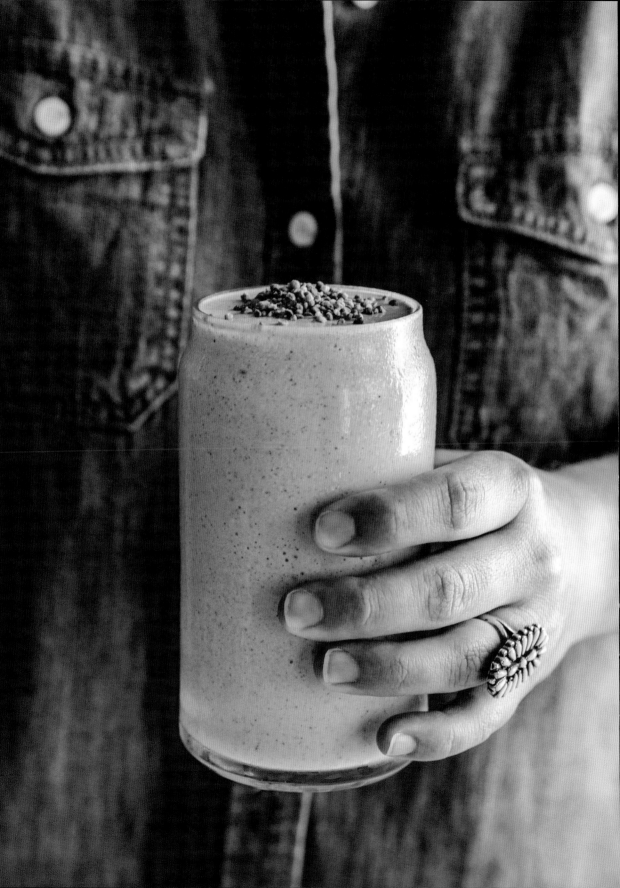

Strawberry Vanilla Almond Butter Smoothie
with Bee Pollen

Research on bee pollen has shown promising reports of antioxidant, anti-inflammatory, anticancer, antibacterial, and immune-enhancing potential—*wow!* Consuming local bee pollen is also thought to increase your immunity to local foliage that typically causes seasonal allergies. And it makes for a fun, colorful, and nutrient-dense addition to your smoothie. SERVES 2

DF | GF | V | Ve

1 cup frozen strawberries

1 frozen peeled banana, halved

1½ cups plain unsweetened plant-based milk or Almond Milk (page 99)

3 tablespoons unsweetened creamy almond butter

1 teaspoon vanilla extract

2–3 pitted dates

Bee pollen (optional)

Add all ingredients, except the bee pollen, to a blender and blend on high until smooth, about 45 to 60 seconds. Pour into individual glasses, top each with a heaping spoonful of bee pollen, and enjoy. Double your recipe or store leftovers (without bee pollen) in the refrigerator in glass jars with airtight lids for 1 to 3 days. After refrigerating, shake well before drinking and top with bee pollen.

> If you are allergic to bee stings or have a history of anaphylaxis from them, do not consume bee pollen, as it may trigger an immune response.

Baby Spinach and Spring Onion Frittata
with Goat Cheese

This frittata is loaded with gorgeous baby spring greens. Spinach is ultra-rich in magnesium and iron and contains healthy amounts of vitamins B2 and B6 as well. Combined with nutrient-dense eggs, you can't go wrong with this one! If you can't find spring onions at your local market or grocery store, substitute scallions. SERVES 6-8

GF | V

1 tablespoon olive oil

1 bunch spring onions, chopped

4 cups packed baby spinach, chopped

½ teaspoon sea salt, divided

12 eggs

½ cup whole milk

¼ cup finely grated Parmesan cheese

¼ teaspoon ground black pepper

2 ounces plain soft goat cheese

Preheat oven to 350°F. Add the olive oil to a 9- or 10-inch cast iron skillet and heat on medium to high heat. Add the spring onions and sauté until softened and tender, about 1 minute. Remove from the heat; add the spinach and ¼ teaspoon of salt. Using a wooden spoon, stir the spinach in the hot cast iron pan until wilted and softened. Spread the onions and spinach evenly around the pan and set aside.

In a large mixing bowl, add the eggs, milk, Parmesan cheese, ¼ teaspoon salt, and pepper; whisk together until thoroughly combined. Pour the egg mixture over the sautéed onions and spinach and stir using the wooden spoon. The vegetables should be evenly dispersed in the egg mixture. Using your hands, tear small teaspoon-size pieces of goat cheese from the cheese log or container and distribute evenly over the egg mixture in the pan.

Place the pan in the oven and bake for 24 to 26 minutes, or until the edges of the frittata have solidified and the center is slightly jiggly (remember your frittata will continue to cook in the cast iron pan once it's removed from the oven). You do not want to overcook the frittata, or it will become spongy and rubbery. Remove from the oven and serve immediately. Store leftovers in an airtight container in the refrigerator for 3 to 4 days. Reheat individual servings when you're ready to eat.

> Frittatas are extremely diverse and accepting of a variety of seasonal vegetables and greens. Use what you have on hand. Remember, though, to sauté any vegetables before adding the eggs for ideal texture and tenderness.

Butter-Roasted Radishes with Radish Greens

In my second trimester of pregnancy, I *may* have eaten this entire dish by myself in one sitting. What can I say?! They're that good. Did you know that radishes are classified as a cruciferous vegetable? Cool fact: you can actually increase the nutrient contribution of all cruciferous veggies (radishes, broccoli, cauliflower, brussel sprouts, etc.) by letting them sit out for several minutes after chopping them, which in turn increases their enzymatic activity and potency. SERVES 4

GF | V

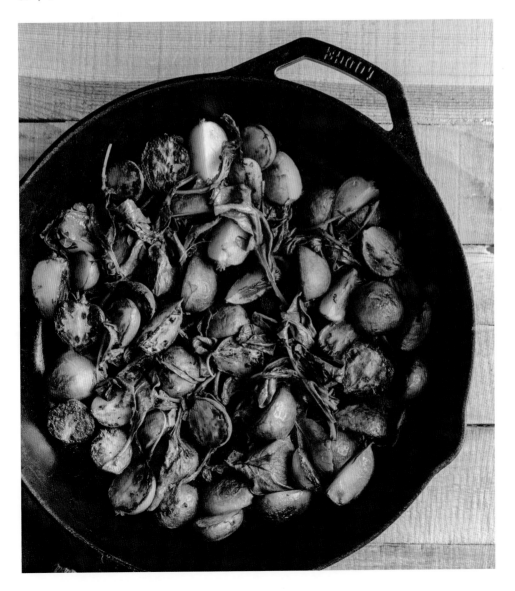

2 bunches radishes with
    greens attached

1 tablespoon butter

¼ teaspoon sea salt

½ small lemon

Preheat oven to 450°F. Remove the radish greens from each radish at the bottom of the stem where they attach to the radish. There's no need to remove the stem nub or the root tail (I personally like the way they look when left on), but feel free to do so if you prefer. Wash and dry the radishes and greens thoroughly. Leave the greens whole and set aside. Halve each radish lengthwise from stem to root, unless your radishes are very small.

Heat the butter in a cast iron skillet or large sauté pan over high heat until bubbling and hot. Place the halved radishes, flat side down, in the skillet and sauté until browned and slightly blistered, about 1 minute. Depending on the size of your skillet, you may need to cook them in two batches. Once all the radishes are browned, return them all to the skillet, with either side facing up, and place the skillet in the oven to roast for 10 minutes.

Remove the hot pan from the oven and set on a heat-resistant surface or stovetop (with heat turned off). Be careful as the skillet is extremely hot! Immediately add the radish greens and salt, sautéing the greens in the oven-hot pan with the residual butter and roasted radishes. Toss with metal tongs for about 1 minute, or until the greens are softened and reduce in size. Finally, squeeze half a lemon over the radishes and greens and give everything one final toss before serving hot directly from the skillet.

Sautéed Fiddlehead Ferns
with Garlic Butter

Fiddlehead ferns are one of spring's wild delicacies. If you're lucky enough to get your hands on some in the short seasonal window, you'll be happy to know these cool-looking coils are packed with vitamin A, vitamin C, and iron, as well as other powerful minerals and electrolytes for optimal health. Consider substituting seasonal spring asparagus if you can't find fiddleheads at your local grocery store or farmer's market. SERVES 3-4

GF | V

1 pound fiddlehead ferns (about 2½ cups) (see note)

2 tablespoons butter

4 garlic cloves, minced

1 tablespoon fish sauce

> Never eat raw fiddleheads. Boil or steam them before consuming. There have been reports of headaches, nausea, and diarrhea from eating fiddleheads that were not adequately cooked.

Thoroughly clean and trim the fiddleheads. Bring a large pot of water to a boil and add the fiddleheads, cooking for 10 minutes. Remove from the heat, drain the water, and set aside.

Melt the butter in a large cast iron skillet over high heat. Sauté the fiddleheads for about 2 minutes with minimal stirring until they're blistered and begin to brown on one side. Sauté for 1 additional minute, stirring constantly. Finally, add the garlic and sauté for 30 more seconds before adding the fish sauce; cook until all the liquid evaporates, about 1 minute. Remove from the heat and serve warm.

Vegetable Miso Soup
with Kombu Dashi and Tofu

The health benefits of this soup are fantastic and can be attributed to the variety of nutrient-dense vegetables, plant-based protein, medicinal mushrooms, mineral-rich seaweed, and probiotic-packed miso. And the kombu dashi makes this recipe sing! Dashi is a traditional Japanese soup stock made in a variety of different ways using a few quality ingredients such as kombu seaweed and/or bonito (a type of fish) flakes. Omit the dashi and just use water if you prefer. SERVES 8

DF | GF | V | Ve

Two 1" × 4" pieces dried kombu seaweed

6 cups water

1 tablespoon toasted sesame oil

2 large carrots, peeled and halved lengthwise, sliced thin

2 celery stalks, sliced thin crosswise

¼ head green cabbage (about 2 cups), cored and chopped into bite-size pieces

2 tablespoons grated ginger

1 tablespoon plus 1 teaspoon soy sauce or gluten-free tamari

2 cloves garlic, grated or minced

⅓ cup plus 2 tablespoons white miso paste

8 ounces firm tofu, drained and gently cut into ½-inch cubes

2 tablespoons dried wakame seaweed

2–3 ounces (1 small handful) fresh enoki mushrooms

¼ cup chopped scallions

Start by making the kombu dashi. Skip this step if you're only using water. In a Dutch oven, combine the kombu and water; bring to a gentle simmer over low heat for 10 to 15 minutes. Do not boil the dashi or the seaweed will impart a bitter taste. Remove from the heat and strain the dashi into a large bowl, discarding the kombu pieces. Set aside.

In the same Dutch oven, heat the oil on medium heat. Add the carrots, celery, cabbage, ginger, and soy sauce, and sauté for 4 to 5 minutes until the vegetables are tender. Add the garlic and sauté for an additional 30 to 60 seconds or until fragrant.

In a small bowl, whisk together the miso paste and 1 cup of the kombu dashi. Add the miso/dashi mixture to the vegetables, along with the remaining 5 cups of kombu dashi, and stir to combine. Next, add the tofu, wakame, mushrooms, and scallions; mix well. Heat the soup on low to medium heat or until hot (not boiling) and ready to serve, about 15 to 20 minutes. The wakame will need at least 15 minutes to fully rehydrate and soften. Enjoy!

Spicy Sriracha Mung Bean Bowl
with Pickled Daikon and Carrots

This is a choose-your-own adventure meal that allows you to customize your bowl however you like and a great meal for batch cooking (see page 116). The rice and beans create a winning combination called a "complete protein" or "complementing proteins." This means that together they supply all nine essential amino acids—the protein building blocks that are especially important in a vegetarian or vegan diet. Contemporary research shows that as long as you eat complete proteins over the course of one to two days, you can attain adequate amounts of these essential amino acids. Read more about complete proteins on page 32.

SERVES 8-10

GF | V | Ve

GRAIN/BEAN BASE

2 cups short-grain brown rice

6½ cups water, divided

1 cup dried mung beans or sprouted dried mung beans

PICKLES

¾ cup shredded orange carrot (about 1 large carrot)

¾ cup shredded daikon radish (about ½ large radish)

¾ cup white wine vinegar

3 tablespoons honey or maple syrup

¾ teaspoon sea salt

SALAD

3 cups chopped napa cabbage (about 1 small head)

1 cup chopped red cabbage (about ¼ medium head)

½ cucumber, sliced lengthwise and chopped into thin sticks

4 scallions, chopped

1 tablespoon toasted sesame oil

1 tablespoon rice wine vinegar

Pinch of sea salt

> If you're planning ahead, soak the brown rice for at least 8 hours or overnight and the mung beans (separately) for at least 12 hours in water. Drain and rinse both before cooking. If you're using sprouted dried mung beans, it's not necessary to soak them ahead of time.

Add the rice and 3½ cups of the water to a small saucepan; bring to a boil over high heat. If you're using soaked rice, use only 3 cups of the water. Once it's boiling, reduce the heat to a simmer and cover with a lid, cooking the rice until it's light and fluffy, about 45 to 50 minutes. If you're using soaked rice, reduce the cooking time. The rice should absorb all the water once it's done cooking, but always taste-test for the optimal texture. Remove from the heat and take off the lid. This will yield about 6 cups of cooked rice.

Prepare the mung beans by placing the beans in a large saucepan with enough water to cover them completely, about 2½ cups. Heat on high heat until boiling, then reduce the heat to a simmer and cover. Cook the beans for about 1 hour or until tender. If you're using soaked beans, reduce the cooking time. Drain the cooked beans and set aside. If you're using sprouted dried mung beans, follow the instructions on the package, as the cooking method and time vary greatly.

→

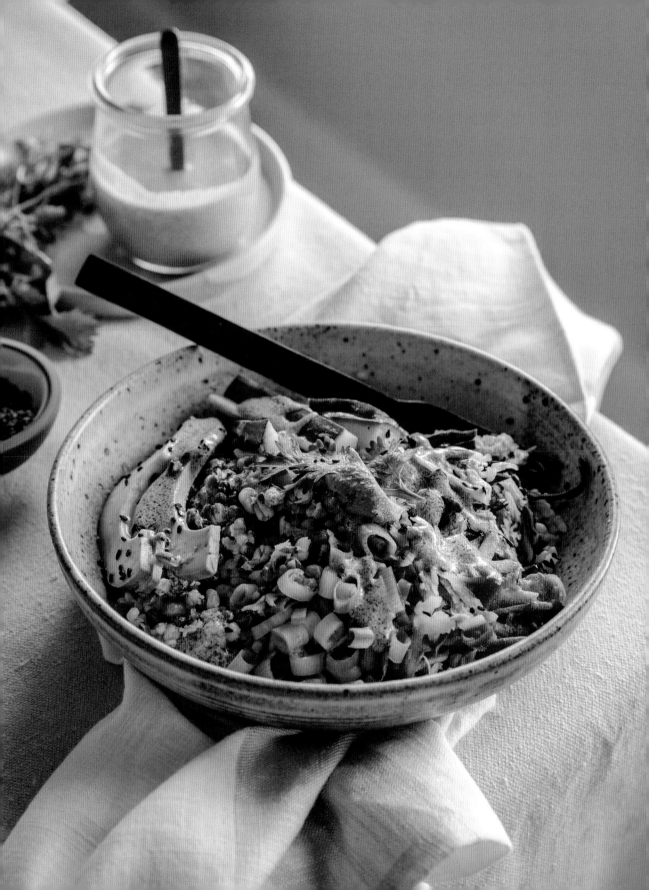

⅓ cup plain sour cream, whole
  milk yogurt, or plant-based
  alternative

3 tablespoons sriracha

1 tablespoon red wine vinegar

¼ teaspoon garlic powder

¼ teaspoon sea salt

⅓ cup avocado oil

TOPPINGS

1 avocado, sliced

Cilantro, chopped

Black sesame seeds

Next, make the pickles. Add the shredded carrot and daikon to a 1-quart glass jar and set aside. Put the vinegar, honey or maple syrup, and salt in a small saucepan over medium heat and stir until all ingredients are dissolved and fully incorporated. Do not boil. Pour the hot vinegar solution over the carrot/daikon mixture in the jar and set on the counter to cool to room temperature before adding the lid and refrigerating. Ideally, these should be fully cooled before eating for optimal flavor, but room temperature carrot/daikon pickles are good too.

Time to prepare the salad. In a large bowl, combine all salad ingredients and toss thoroughly. Set aside. To prepare the dressing, place all ingredients except the avocado oil in a high-powered blender and blend on high. Once all the ingredients are combined, slowly drizzle in the oil, keeping the blender on, until the dressing is thick and smooth. Lastly, prepare the toppings and set aside.

Finally, it's time for assembly. Build your bowl however you like! Layer a serving of cooked rice and beans on the bottom of a serving bowl. Add a handful of salad and a heaping spoonful of pickles. Dress the entire bowl with the desired amount of dressing and finish with your favorite toppings. You can customize a bowl to order for each person and/or each meal. Serve this salad at room temperature or chilled. Store each component separately in the refrigerator for 3 to 4 days for optimal freshness. The pickles will last up to 6 months in the refrigerator and the dressing can be stored for 5 to 7 days.

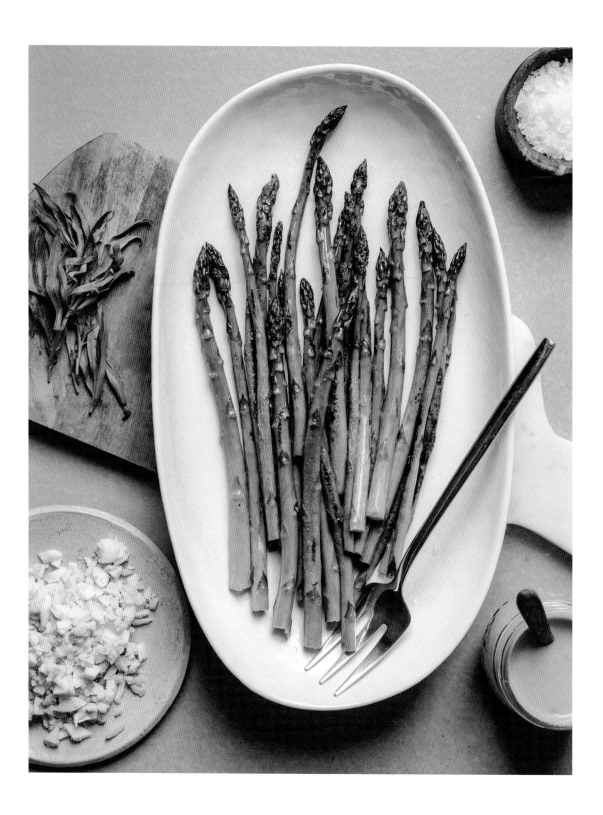

Grilled Asparagus Salad
with Chopped Eggs and Tarragon Vinaigrette

This is an homage to a beloved French dish called *asperges mimosa* (asparagus mimosa), which means "asparagus garnished with egg yolk"—and that's just what we do! Eggs are a fantastic source of protein, omega-3 fatty acids, vitamin E, choline, selenium, and many other worthy nutrients. Also, did you know that if you have healthy blood cholesterol levels, there's no need to avoid eggs as was previously thought? In several large-scale studies, people who ate one to six eggs per week showed no health risks and, in fact, had increased levels of HDL, or "good cholesterol." Just remember to choose organic, pastured, humanely-raised eggs whenever possible. SERVES 2-3

DF | GF | V

2 eggs

2 shallots, peeled

1 tablespoon Dijon mustard

2 tablespoons fresh tarragon, divided

1 tablespoon sherry vinegar

¾ teaspoon sea salt, divided

¼ cup plus 3 teaspoons olive oil, divided

1 bunch asparagus (about 12–14 spears)

2 tablespoons chopped flat-leaf parsley

Preheat a grill to high heat. Alternatively, you can use a cast iron grill pan on your stovetop. Add the eggs to a small saucepan and cover with 1 to 2 inches of water. Bring the water and eggs to a boil over high heat. Once the water is boiling, turn off heat, but leave the pan on the burner, and cover. Let it sit for 12 minutes, then remove the pan from the stove and run cold water into it until the eggs and water are cool. Peel and dice the eggs into small pieces and set aside.

To make the dressing, add the shallots, mustard, 1 tablespoon tarragon, vinegar, and ¼ teaspoon salt to a high-powered blender. Blend until smooth, about 30 seconds. Slowly drizzle in ¼ cup olive oil, with the blender on, until the dressing is emulsified. Season to taste and pour the finished dressing into a small jar or pitcher; set aside.

Trim off approximately the bottom quarter of each asparagus spear. Place the asparagus on a small baking sheet or half sheet pan, and add 3 teaspoons olive oil and ½ teaspoon salt. Use clean hands to toss and coat the spears. Place the asparagus directly on the preheated grill or grill pan, perpendicular to the grating. Grill for 10 to 15 minutes with the lid open, or in your grill pan, exposing all sides to the heat to evenly brown. Remove the asparagus from the grill or pan and put directly on a serving dish.

Pour the dressing over the asparagus and sprinkle with the diced eggs, 1 tablespoon tarragon, and the parsley. Serve warm or at room temperature.

Chicken Meatballs
with Basil Walnut Pesto

These meatballs are inspired by Julia Turshen's Turkey + Ricotta Meatballs recipe from her cookbook *Small Victories*, and they are super simple and satisfying to make—a leaner version of a traditional beef or pork meatball. I like to serve them warm as an appetizer with toothpicks and the pesto as a dipping sauce or tossed in the pesto with whole wheat spaghetti noodles as part of my meal. Also, they're tasty served cold on top of a hearty green salad or eaten straight from the fridge! MAKES ABOUT 26 MEATBALLS AND ABOUT ¼ CUP PESTO

GF

MEATBALLS

2 pounds ground dark meat chicken (or a mixture of white and dark meat)

1 cup whole milk ricotta

4 cloves garlic, minced

⅓ cup finely chopped parsley

⅓ cup finely chopped basil

1 tablespoon sea salt

Olive oil

PESTO

2 cups fresh basil

2 garlic cloves

¼ cup walnuts, toasted and cooled

¼ cup grated Parmesan cheese

½ teaspoon sea salt

½ cup olive oil

Preheat oven to 425°F. Add all meatball ingredients except the olive oil to a large mixing bowl, and mix together with a fork or clean hands until thoroughly combined. Roll the mixture into medium-size (about 1½-inch) balls and place evenly on a baking sheet brushed with olive oil. It's OK if they're soft and not perfectly round (this translates to tender meatballs that look handmade and more authentic). Brush each meatball lightly with olive oil; bake for 25 to 30 minutes until lightly browned and cooked through. Remove from the oven and set aside.

While the meatballs are baking, make the pesto. Add all pesto ingredients, except for the olive oil, to a small food processor and process until finely minced and almost a paste. Stop to scrape down the sides. Continue running the food processor and slowly drizzle olive oil into the mixture—or add 1 tablespoon at a time, pulsing in between—until the pesto comes together and is smooth.

Place the meatballs and pesto in a large bowl and toss until the meatballs are fully coated, or place the meatballs on a plate and spoon pesto over each one. Sprinkle with additional Parmesan cheese if desired. Serve warm or refrigerate and serve cold. Keep the leftovers in an airtight container in the refrigerator for 3 to 4 days or freeze (cooked) meatballs and the pesto separately for up to 6 months.

Vegetable Fried Brown Rice
with Ginger Sauce

Brown rice is a more nutrient-dense option than its white counterpart because it includes the grain in its whole form with all of its edible parts—bran, germ, and endosperm. Including all of these classifies it as a whole grain. With eight different vegetables and a whole grain, this recipe provides plentiful fiber, antioxidants, vitamins, and minerals. Remember, too, that the best fried rice should take mere minutes to cook. To achieve this, you must prepare all of your ingredients ahead of time (aka prepare a *mise en place*) and use a very hot pan. SERVES 8

DF | GF | V | Ve

1 cup uncooked) long-grain brown rice

1¾ cups water

3 garlic cloves, minced

1 tablespoon finely grated ginger

¼ cup gluten-free tamari or soy sauce

2 tablespoons mirin

1 tablespoon chili oil

3 teaspoons toasted sesame oil, divided

1 cup chopped white onion

1 cup chopped carrots

1 cup thinly sliced red cabbage

1 cup chopped red bell pepper

2 cups broccoli florets

1 cup frozen green peas, thawed and drained

1 cup sliced shiitake mushrooms, stems removed

2 eggs or 6 ounces extra-firm tofu

3 scallions, chopped

Sesame seeds

> Use leftover rice or cook and cool fresh rice on a baking sheet ahead of time to ensure drier, stickier rice kernels for the optimal fried rice texture. If you're making fresh rice and planning ahead, soak the uncooked rice in water for at least 8 hours or overnight. Drain the rice and rinse before cooking.

Start by making the rice. Add the uncooked brown rice and water to a small saucepan and bring to a boil over high heat. If you're using soaked rice, use only 1½ cups water. Once boiling, reduce the heat to a simmer and cover with a lid, cooking the rice until it's light and fluffy, about 45 to 50 minutes. If you're using soaked rice, reduce the cooking time. The rice should absorb all the water once it's done cooking, but always taste-test for the optimal texture. Remove from the heat and immediately take off the lid. This will yield about 3½ cups of cooked rice. Spread the rice evenly on a baking sheet and let cool.

In a small bowl, whisk together the garlic, ginger, tamari, mirin, and chili oil; set aside. If you don't like spicy chili oil, you can omit it and replace with additional toasted sesame oil instead.

In a large wok or cast iron skillet on the stovetop, heat 1½ teaspoons sesame oil over high heat. Add the onion, carrots, and cabbage; using a wooden spoon, stir-fry for 2 to 3 minutes until browned and crisp. Quickly remove the vegetables from the wok and set aside. Add the remaining 1½ teaspoons of sesame oil, the bell pepper, broccoli, peas, and mushrooms to the wok; stir-fry for 1 to 2 minutes. Remove the vegetables and set aside.

→

You can substitute almost any vegetable in this dish, just consider their moisture content. Too much moisture will create a soggier fried rice, which is less than ideal.

Crack the eggs or crumble the tofu into the hot wok or skillet (adding more oil if necessary), and scramble or mix around with your wooden spoon until just cooked through, about 60 seconds. Add the rice and ginger sauce and stir together until the rice is fully coated, breaking up any chunks as necessary.

Add all the previously cooked vegetables and stir together until thoroughly combined. Remove from the heat and top with scallions and sesame seeds. Serve hot.

Creamy "Alfredo" Pasta
with Roasted Broccoli and Baby Kale

The creamy texture of the sauce comes from cauliflower—the perfect, nutrient-dense alternative to a rich and traditional alfredo sauce. You can easily make this recipe gluten-free, dairy-free, and/or vegan. I prefer whole wheat linguine or fettuccine noodles with butter and Parmesan cheese, but feel free to substitute with alternative versions to meet your dietary needs. SERVES 6

V | GF

1 pound broccoli (about 1 head), cut into small florets

3 teaspoons olive oil

1 teaspoon sea salt, divided

1 pound dried pasta of choice

4 cups vegetable stock

2 pounds cauliflower (about 1 head), cut into 8 pieces

2 tablespoons unsalted butter

4 cloves garlic, minced

½ cup finely grated Parmesan cheese

1½ cups baby kale, destemmed

Preheat oven to 425°F. Spread the broccoli florets on a baking sheet and toss with olive oil and ¼ teaspoon salt. Roast broccoli for 15 to 20 minutes until fork tender and slightly crispy. Remove from oven and set aside.

Prepare your pasta of choice, following the cooking instructions on the package. Once it's done cooking, drain off the water and set the noodles aside.

In a Dutch oven or large saucepan on high heat, bring the vegetable stock to a boil. Add the cauliflower pieces and cover with a lid; continue to boil, steaming the cauliflower for 8 to 10 minutes or until fork tender. In a small saucepan, melt the butter on low to medium heat; add the garlic and lightly sauté for 30 to 60 seconds or until fragrant. Do not burn the garlic or it will become bitter.

Remove the cauliflower from the vegetable stock using a slotted spoon and place it in a blender with 1¼ cups of the vegetable stock. Reserve the remaining stock and set aside. Add the sautéed butter and garlic and blend on high until completely puréed and silky smooth, about 1 to 2 minutes. The cauliflower purée should be thick, yet smooth and pourable like a traditional alfredo sauce. Add more vegetable stock to thin the sauce if needed. This is the base for your sauce.

Transfer the "alfredo" sauce to the original Dutch oven and stir in the cheese and ¾ teaspoon salt. Bring the sauce to a low simmer, stirring regularly to keep it from burning, while the cheese melts. Once the cheese is fully incorporated, add the roasted broccoli, cooked noodles, and fresh kale, and heat all the ingredients together on low to medium heat until the pasta and broccoli are heated through and the kale is wilted, about 5 minutes. Add more vegetable stock if needed. Season to taste. Serve warm topped with additional grated Parmesan if desired.

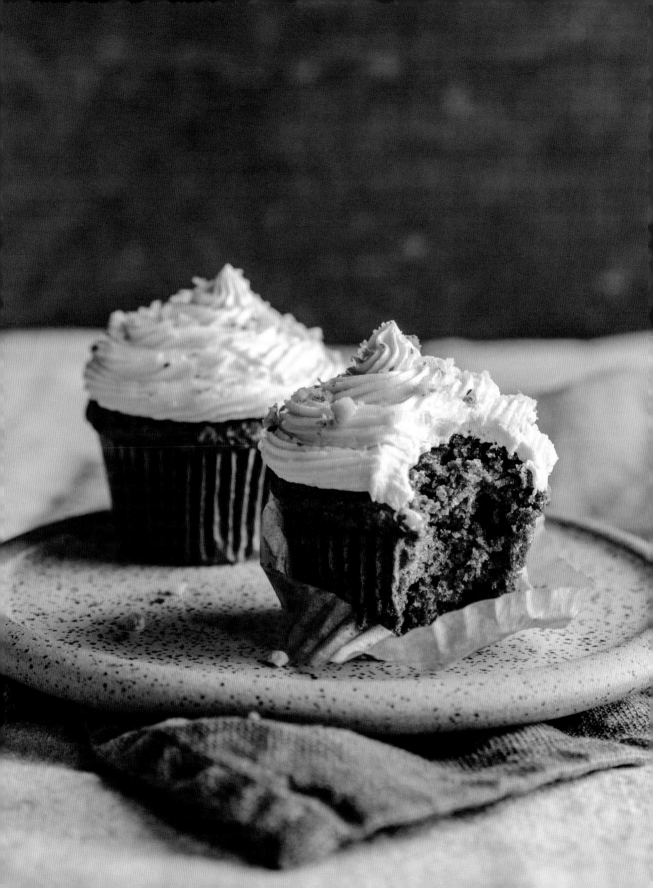

Carrot Cake Cupcakes with Vanilla Tofu Frosting

These cupcakes are dairy-free, and refined sugar-free—a fantastic recipe for every day or any special occasion like baby's first birthday. You'll be happy to know that each cupcake delivers a substantial serving of protein and fiber. The tofu frosting is a cool twist on a traditional vanilla buttercream, but you can easily substitute buttercream or cream cheese frosting if preferred. **MAKES 12 CUPCAKES**

DF | V

CUPCAKES

1¾ cup whole wheat pastry flour

2 teaspoons baking soda

1 teaspoon sea salt

2½ teaspoons ground cinnamon

½ teaspoon ground ginger

½ teaspoon ground cloves

½ teaspoon ground nutmeg

½ cup walnut oil

½ cup honey

3 eggs, whisked

¾ cup unsweetened applesauce

4 large carrots, finely grated (about 1½ cups)

TOFU FROSTING

12–14 ounces firm or extra-firm tofu

¼ cup honey

2 tablespoons unsweetened creamy almond butter

1½ teaspoons vanilla extract

1 vanilla bean pod or ½ teaspoon vanilla bean paste

OPTIONAL GARNISHES

½ cup finely chopped walnuts

1 large carrot, finely grated with zester or fine grater

Ground cinnamon

Preheat oven to 350°F. Line a muffin pan with paper muffin cups and set aside.

In a large mixing bowl, mix together the flour, baking soda, salt, and spices; set aside. Add the oil, honey, eggs, and applesauce to a clean, large mixing bowl and whisk together until fully incorporated. Add the wet ingredients to the dry ingredients and mix with a wooden spoon until just combined. Be careful not to overmix your batter (it's OK if there are some small bits of flour not mixed in). Fold in the grated carrots until evenly incorporated.

Spoon the muffin batter into muffin cups, filling each to the top. Bake for 22 to 24 minutes or until a toothpick inserted in the center of a muffin comes out clean. Remove from the oven and cool the muffin pan on a wire rack for at least 10 minutes, or until the muffins are completely cooled. While the cupcakes are cooling, make the frosting.

Add all frosting ingredients except the vanilla pod to a blender (if using vanilla bean paste, you can add it now). Split the vanilla pod in half lengthwise and scrape out the beans with the backside of a knife. Add them to the blender and blend on high until the mixture is smooth and creamy, but not runny, about 2 to 3 minutes. Add more nut butter if you want "stiffer" frosting, especially if you're planning to pipe decorations on the cupcakes. Store the frosting in the refrigerator in an airtight container until ready to use. Frosting will keep for about 3 days before it will begin to separate.

Now you're ready for assembly! Frost each cooled cupcake generously with frosting using a knife or a pastry bag with a decorative tip. Sprinkle with chopped walnuts, finely grated carrot, and a light dusting of cinnamon.

Leftover cupcakes (without frosting) will keep in an airtight container at room temperature for 3 days before drying out. If frosted, you can store the cupcakes in an airtight container in the refrigerator for 1 to 2 days.

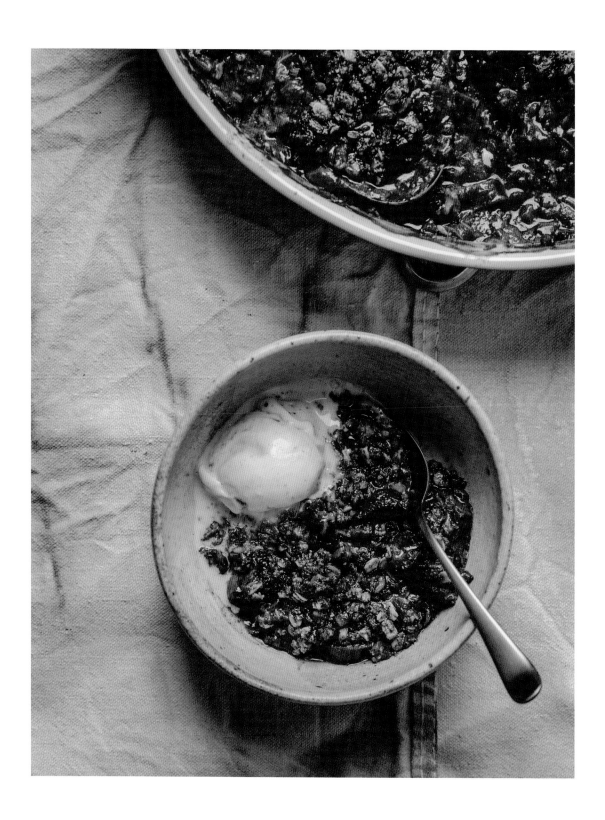

Strawberry Rhubarb Crisp

This old-fashioned dessert is a seasonal celebration of spring's bounty featuring strawberries and rhubarb. The traditional version gets a slight makeover by replacing wheat flour with almond flour, making this a great gluten-free dessert. If you can't find superfine almond flour, look for "almond meal," which is also just ground almonds but typically with a coarser grind. Or consider grinding your own, using whole almonds and a quality food processor or high-powered blender. SERVES 9

DF | GF | V | Ve

1 pound strawberries, hulled and chopped

½ pound rhubarb, chopped

¼ cup honey or maple syrup

2 teaspoons vanilla extract

1 tablespoon arrowroot powder

1 cup rolled oats

⅔ cup superfine almond flour (natural or blanched)

½ cup Sucanat or coconut sugar

⅓ cup pecans, finely chopped

⅓ cup walnuts, finely chopped

1 teaspoon ground cinnamon

¼ teaspoon ground nutmeg

Pinch of sea salt

6 tablespoons butter or coconut oil, melted

Preheat oven to 350°F. Grease an 8" × 8" baking dish or cast iron skillet, and set aside.

In a large mixing bowl, mix the strawberries, rhubarb, honey, and vanilla extract well. Add the arrowroot powder and stir to combine. In a separate large mixing bowl, mix together the rolled oats, almond flour, sugar, nuts, spices, and salt. Pour the melted butter or coconut oil into the bowl with the oat mixture and, using a fork, stir together until it resembles coarse crumbs.

Add the fruit mixture to the greased pan or skillet, and top with the oat mixture. Make sure the oat mixture is spread evenly over the fruit layer so it bakes evenly. Bake for 35 to 45 minutes until the fruit is tender and the juices are bubbling. Remove from the oven; let cool slightly before serving with a scoop of vanilla ice cream or plain yogurt.

Store any leftovers in the refrigerator, lightly covered but not completely sealed, to preserve the topping's texture, for 4 to 5 days. Remove cover and reheat in the oven at 350°F.

7
SUMMER

Summer is a joyous and expansive season reflected in the sun and the energy of an exploding garden. We are empowered and excited during this season and fully embodied. We gather together communally and effortlessly to celebrate our vitality.

Our appetite decreases as our digestive efficiency builds. We transition to a mostly fresh and raw plant-based diet with ease. We thrive on the abundant and cooling vegetables and hydrating, sweet fruits the season has to offer. Fresh produce, plant proteins, whole grains, some dairy, and sea vegetables find their way to our plates. We treasure each cucumber, pepper, tomato, corn kernel, stone fruit, and berry that grows in abundance.

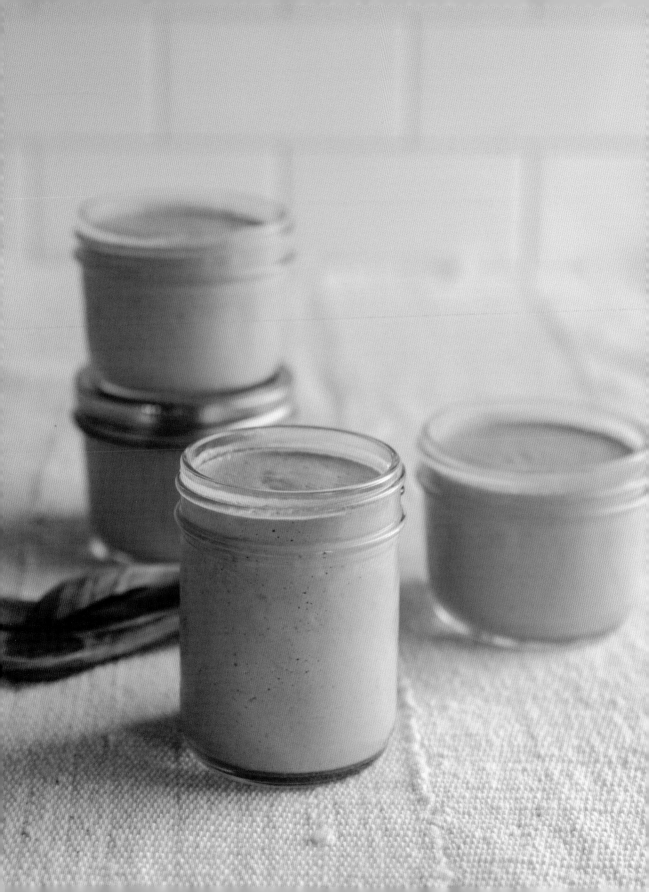

Cultured Key Lime Cashew Yogurt

You'll feel like a magician after making this probiotic-rich vegan yogurt! For something so easy, the outcome is complex and incredibly healthy, especially for your gut. Probiotics have been shown to support a healthy digestive tract while also boosting the immune system, lowering blood pressure, helping to manage anxiety, and so much more! If you can't find key limes at your local grocery store or farmer's market, you can easily substitute conventional (Persian) limes. MAKES FOUR 8-OUNCE JARS

DF | GF | V | Ve | RT

2 cups raw cashews, soaked for at least 1 hour or overnight

1½ cups unsweetened plain cashew milk or other plant-based milk

5 tablespoons maple syrup

2 tablespoons key lime or Persian lime zest (about 16 key limes or 3 Persian limes)

½ cup fresh key lime or Persian lime juice (about 16 key limes or 3 Persian limes)

3 tablespoons packed kale or spinach (fresh or frozen)

Probiotic capsules or powder (see note)

There are many types of probiotics, including different bacterial strains, doses or amounts of colony forming units (CFUs), and forms. Here, you'll want to use a total of 20 to 30 billion CFUs of a lactobacillus blend in either capsule or powder form (read the label). If you use less than this, you won't get that tangy yogurt flavor, and the texture will be slightly looser or thinner. More, and your yogurt will become really sour and may be unappealing.

Drain and rinse the cashews. Place the cashews, milk, and maple syrup in a blender; blend on high until very smooth with no lumps, about 1 to 2 minutes if you're using a high-powered blender. If you want plain cashew yogurt, you can omit the lime and move on to the next step. Or you can substitute other fresh seasonal juice/flavors, if you prefer, such as orange or passion fruit.

Zest your limes and set the zest aside. Add the lime juice and kale or spinach (for a subtle green color) to your blender; blend on high until puréed and smooth. Pour into a large mixing bowl and add the lime zest, stirring with a rubber spatula until incorporated.

Finally, add the probiotics to the cashew blend and whisk in thoroughly. Divide the cashew yogurt evenly between four 8-ounce glass jars. Place small squares of cheesecloth or paper towel over the jars; screw on the metal jar rings or use rubber bands to secure the cheesecloth. Do not use the full lid at this point; you want some air flow into the jar. Once all the jars are assembled, arrange them on a baking sheet and place in the oven, with the heat off and the oven light on, near the oven light for residual low heat. Let the yogurt incubate in the oven for at least 8 hours or overnight. The longer you leave it, the tangier and thicker it becomes.

Remove the jars and the cheesecloth or paper towel, and seal the jars completely with airtight lids. Refrigerate for at least 1 hour or more until chilled and ready to serve. Yogurt will keep in the refrigerator for about 7 days. Stir each yogurt before serving—natural separation may occur after one to two days.

Egg Muffins

with Tomato Salsa and Lime-Marinated Avocado

These super satisfying egg muffins are customizable for a variety of tastes and diets. The avocado in this version provides healthy fat and is a great source of fiber, as well as multiple vitamins and minerals. To get the most phytonutrients possible, cut your avocado in half and peel each half with your hands, preserving as much of the dark green outermost flesh closest to the peel as possible. MAKES 12 EGG MUFFINS

GF | V

Avocado oil

12 eggs

¾ teaspoon sea salt, divided

½ teaspoon ground black pepper

½ cup finely chopped yellow onion (about ½ medium onion)

½ cup diced red bell pepper (about ½ red bell pepper)

½ cup diced green bell pepper (about ½ green bell pepper)

¼ cup chopped fresh cilantro

¼ cup grated cheddar cheese

Juice of 1 lime

1 tablespoon avocado oil

Pinch of red chili flakes

1 avocado, sliced thin

Tomato salsa

Preheat oven to 350°F. Liberally oil a muffin pan and set aside. Do not line with paper muffin cups.

In a large mixing bowl, whisk the eggs, ½ teaspoon salt, and ground pepper until light and fluffy, about 30 to 60 seconds. In a small mixing bowl, combine the onions and bell peppers. Distribute the vegetable mixture evenly between the 12 muffin cups. Using a large spoon or ¼-cup measuring scoop, add the egg mixture to each muffin cup until evenly divided. Top each with cilantro and cheese. Bake for 18 to 20 minutes, or until the muffins start to rise and are cooked through. There should be no egg liquid left on the surface of the muffins.

While the muffins are baking, marinate the avocado. In a small bowl, whisk the lime juice, avocado oil, ¼ teaspoon salt, and chili flakes together. Add the avocado slices to the marinade, stirring gently to coat each piece evenly; set aside until ready to serve.

Once the egg muffins are done baking, remove from the oven. Serve the muffins hot, topped with a spoonful of salsa and a slice or two of marinated avocado.

Sweet Cornmeal Pancakes
with Vanilla Roasted Peaches

These are not your mama's pancakes! They are a 100 percent whole grain and gluten-free alternative to a traditional American pancake using all-purpose flour. The cornmeal and oat flour provide more nutrients and ample fiber while delivering a fantastic flavor and heartier pancake similar to a Johnnycake (pancake-like cornmeal patties). Feel free to use any variety of seasonal fruit you have on hand, fresh or roasted and caramelized in the oven. MAKES ABOUT 10 PANCAKES

DF | GF | V | Ve

1½ cups whole grain oat flour

1 cup medium-grind whole grain yellow cornmeal

2 teaspoons baking powder

½ teaspoon sea salt

2 eggs

½ cup whole milk or plant-based alternative

2 tablespoons maple syrup (plus more for serving)

1 cup pitted and sliced peaches (about 2 small peaches)

2 tablespoons salted butter or coconut oil, divided (plus more for serving)

½ teaspoon vanilla extract

In a large mixing bowl, thoroughly mix together the dry ingredients. In a separate medium-size bowl, whisk the eggs until light and fluffy. Add the milk and maple syrup, and whisk together until combined. Add the egg mixture to the dry ingredients and mix until incorporated (I like to use a fork). If there are a few lumps, that's OK. Let the batter sit untouched for 5 minutes. This gives the cornmeal and oat flour time to soak up some of the liquid and thicken the batter slightly. The consistency of your batter should be similar to traditional pancake batter—pourable yet slightly thick. Add more milk to thin or more oat flour to thicken if necessary.

Meanwhile, preheat the oven to 400°F. Line a baking sheet with parchment paper and set aside. In a medium-size bowl, combine the peach slices, 1 tablespoon melted butter or coconut oil, and the vanilla extract. Stir together until the fruit is evenly coated. Spread the peach slices on the baking sheet and roast in the oven for 10 minutes. Remove from the oven, and using a fork, turn all the peach slices. Roast for an additional 10 minutes or until lightly golden. Remove from the oven and set aside. Alternatively, you can halve your peaches, toss them with the butter or coconut oil and vanilla extract , and grill them, cut side down, until golden and caramelized, about 3 to 5 minutes; then slice.

→

Heat your cast iron skillet or griddle to medium heat and melt 1 tablespoon of butter or coconut oil. Using a ¼-cup measuring cup, scoop batter onto the skillet or griddle and cook the first side for about 2 minutes. The underside of the pancake should be a light golden brown before you flip it over. Cook the second side for an additional 1 to 2 minutes, until the pancake is cooked through. Remove from the pan or skillet and serve immediately, topped with additional butter or coconut oil, maple syrup, and a spoonful of roasted peaches.

Creamy Red Pepper and Tomato Soup
with Basil Oil

This savory vegan soup is perfect for a quick weeknight meal and is sure to tantalize your taste buds. It's full of anti-inflammatory nutrients and antioxidants to support cardiovascular health. Did you know that although popular opinion says that tomatoes, as part of the nightshade family, cause inflammation, research shows that they are actually associated with a decreased risk of inflammation and decreased free radicals or toxins? Grab another bowl before it's gone! SERVES 4–6

DF | GF | V | Ve

SOUP

1 pound tomatoes, halved (I prefer vine-ripened)

2 red bell peppers, halved and seeds removed

½ large white or yellow onion, roughly chopped

3 whole garlic cloves

2 tablespoons olive oil

One 6-ounce can tomato paste

One 13.5-ounce can unsweetened full-fat coconut milk

1 cup water

1 teaspoon paprika

1 teaspoon sea salt

Whole basil leaves (garnish)

BASIL OIL

2 cups basil

¾ cup olive oil

Preheat oven to 400°F. Place the tomatoes, red peppers, onion, and garlic on a baking sheet and drizzle with olive oil. Roast for about 30 minutes or until the vegetables get juicy and soften. Remove from the oven and add the vegetables and their juices to a blender. Add the tomato paste, coconut milk, water, paprika, and salt to the blender and blend everything on high until smooth and creamy, about 45 seconds. Pour the blended soup into a Dutch oven or saucepan and warm over medium to high heat until heated through.

Meanwhile, make the basil oil. Process the basil and olive oil in a blender on high until smooth, about 30 to 60 seconds. Lay a double layer of cheesecloth over an 8-ounce glass jar and strain the basil oil into it, squeezing the contents and removing any solids or plant matter in the cheesecloth. Dress individual bowls of hot soup with a small spoonful of basil oil (I like to make a decorative swirl!) and a whole leaf or two of fresh basil. Enjoy this soup with a slice of crusty bread. Alternatively, you can serve this soup cold if you prefer.

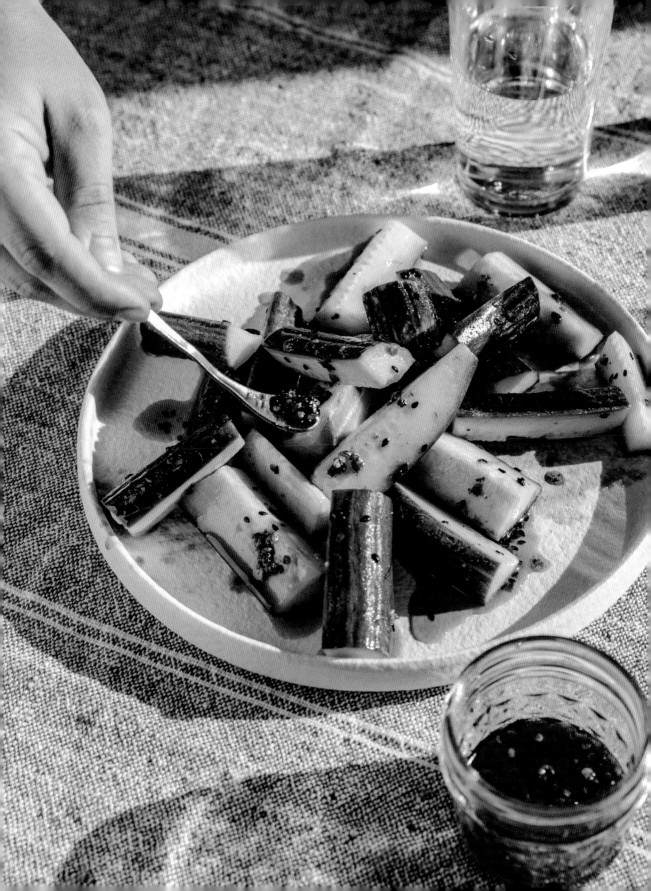

Cucumber Salad
with Honey Sesame Dressing

Cucumbers provide beneficial phytonutrients—specifically carotenoids, flavonoids, and antioxidants—mostly from the skin and seeds, so try to include both whenever you can in recipes calling for cucumbers. Depending on the size of your cucumbers and how ripe they are, the skin should be tender and the seeds small and palatable. SERVES 4-6

DF | GF | V | Ve

2 tablespoons rice wine vinegar

1 tablespoon soy sauce or gluten-free tamari

1 tablespoon toasted sesame oil

1 tablespoon honey or maple syrup

2 teaspoons chili oil (I prefer chili oil that includes pieces of chili)

2 large cucumbers, quartered lengthwise and cut into 3-inch pieces

1 teaspoon black sesame seeds

In a large mixing bowl, whisk together the vinegar, soy sauce or tamari, sesame oil, honey or maple syrup, and chili oil. Add the cucumber pieces and sesame seeds to the liquid dressing, and mix together until evenly coated. Refrigerate for at least 20 minutes or until cold. Give it one final stir and top with additional chili oil if you like it spicy, and serve cold.

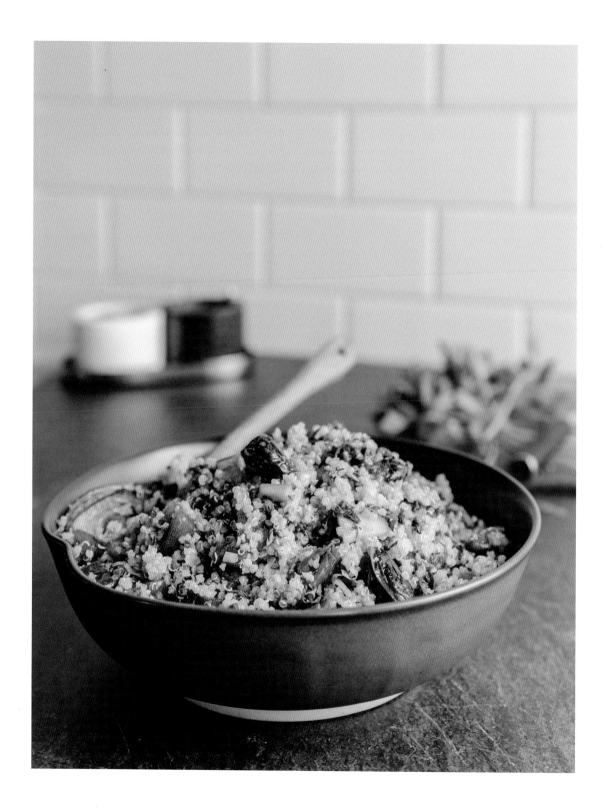

Quinoa Tabbouleh
with Roasted Cherry Tomatoes

Traditional tabbouleh is made with bulgur (a form of wheat), but I like to replace the bulgur with quinoa for more protein and a fun twist on a Middle Eastern classic. The hefty amount of parsley in this recipe provides an excellent source of vitamins C and K and a substantial amount of vitamin A, folate, and iron. Serve on top of a green salad with falafels or alongside grilled vegetables and meat. SERVES 6-8

DF | GF | V | Ve

⅔ cup white quinoa, rinsed and drained

1⅓ cups water

1 pint cherry tomatoes

1 tablespoon plus ⅛ cup olive oil

1¼ teaspoons sea salt, divided

3 medium tomatoes, chopped (about 2½ cups; I prefer vine-ripened or Roma)

1 small cucumber, skin on and seeds included, chopped (about 1 cup)

1 bunch scallions, chopped (about 1 cup)

1 bunch curly parsley, destemmed and chopped (about 2 cups)

¼ cup finely chopped mint

¼ cup lemon juice

> If you're planning ahead, soak the quinoa in water for at least 8 hours or overnight. Drain and rinse before cooking.

Add the quinoa and water to a small saucepan and bring to a boil over high heat. Once it's boiling, reduce the heat to a simmer and cover with a lid; cook the quinoa until it's light and fluffy, about 15 minutes. If you're using soaked quinoa, reduce the cooking time. The quinoa should absorb all the water once it's done cooking, but taste-test for optimal texture. Remove from the heat and carefully spread the hot quinoa evenly on a baking sheet; set aside to cool. This will yield about 2½ cups of cooked quinoa.

Preheat oven to 400°F. In a large bowl, toss the whole cherry tomatoes, 1 tablespoon olive oil, and ¼ teaspoon salt together. Spread on a clean baking sheet and bake for 30 minutes, or until the tomatoes are tender, bubbling, and juicy. Remove from the oven and set aside to cool.

In the same large bowl, add the cooled quinoa, chopped tomatoes, cucumber, scallions, parsley, mint, and cooled cherry tomatoes. In a small bowl, whisk together the lemon juice, ⅛ cup olive oil, and 1 teaspoon salt; pour over the quinoa and stir until the mixture is fully dressed. The tabbouleh should be tangy and herbaceous. Season to taste and serve at room temperature, or refrigerate for 20 to 30 minutes and serve cool.

Salt and Pepper Grilled Prawns
with Chimichurri Corn

This dish screams summer! It's light and oh so flavorful—perfect for eating outside on sunny days and warm nights. Make sure to check with the Monterey Bay Aquarium Seafood Watchlist before shopping for prawns to find the most sustainable option in your area. Read more about sustainable seafood on page 75). SERVES 8

DF | GF

CHIMICHURRI

3 cups flat-leaf parsley

⅓ cup fresh oregano

4 cloves garlic, peeled

2 teaspoons red chili flakes

1 teaspoon sea salt

¼ cup red wine vinegar

½ cup olive oil

CORN AND PRAWNS

8 corn ears, husks and silks removed

2 tablespoons olive oil, divided

24 large or jumbo prawns or shrimp, shelled and deveined, tails intact

¼ teaspoon sea salt

¼ teaspoon ground black pepper

Start by making the chimichurri. Add all ingredients except the olive oil to a food processor and blend until smooth and almost a paste. Transfer the contents to a small bowl and add the olive oil, stirring with a spoon to incorporate. This makes about 2 cups total. Set aside. Chimichurri can be prepared 1 to 2 days in advance and stored in the refrigerator. Bring it to room temperature before serving.

Preheat a grill to medium-high heat. Drizzle a small amount of olive oil (about 1 tablespoon divided between all the ears of corn) on each ear and, and rub it evenly over the corn with clean hands. Place the corn on the grill and close the cover; grill for a total of 15 to 20 minutes, rotating each ear every 5 minutes or so to expose each side to the heat until browned and slightly charred. Using a fork or knife, check to make sure the corn kernels are tender before removing from the heat. Set aside to cool. Once cooled, lay each ear of corn on a cutting board, facing away from you. Run a sharp knife down the long side of the corn cob, slicing off the cooked kernels. Rotate and continue to slice and remove all kernels. Repeat with all the ears. Place the cut kernels into a large mixing bowl and set aside. Alternatively, you can substitute 4 cups frozen corn that you thaw and roast in the oven on high heat with olive oil for 15 to 20 minutes.

Prepare the prawns. In a large bowl, toss the prawns with 1 tablespoon olive oil and salt and pepper to taste. You can use metal or wood skewers. If you're using skewers, thread the prawns on them and place on the grill. Grill the prawns for about 2 minutes on each side or until cooked through. Remove from the heat.

Add the cooked prawns to the mixing bowl with the corn kernels and dress with half (about 1 cup) of the chimichurri to start. Mix together until all ingredients are thoroughly coated with the chimichurri; add more sauce as desired. Place on a large serving dish and serve warm or chill in the refrigerator for 20 minutes before serving.

Rainbow Rolls
with Ginger Almond Sauce

Rainbow chard, a collection of different varieties of chard, is incredibly nutritious, delivering ample amounts of magnesium, iron, manganese, copper, and potassium. Cabbage supports natural detoxification in the body due to its antioxidant content and sulfur-containing compounds. These two powerful plants, combined with the other vegetables, provide a recipe that's abundant in fiber, supports digestive health, and is naturally cleansing. Customize the ingredients to fit your preferred flavor profile, keeping in mind color and textural variation. Add thinly sliced and cooked fish, shrimp, tofu, or a spread of nut butter for more protein if desired. MAKES ABOUT 8 ROLLS AND 1 CUP SAUCE

DF | GF | V | Ve

ROLLS

2 cups dried thin rice noodles or vermicelli rice noodles

Toasted sesame oil

1 bunch rainbow chard, destemmed and each leaf torn in half crosswise

½ small red cabbage, cored and shredded or thinly sliced (about 2 cups)

1 yellow bell pepper, julienned (about 1 cup)

½ English cucumber, seeded and julienned (about ¾ cup)

1 large carrot, peeled and julienned (about ¾ cups)

1 cup cilantro, destemmed (thin stems OK)

Eight (8 inch) spring roll rice paper wrappers

Follow the manufacturer's instructions for cooking the rice noodles. Once they are cooked, drain the softened noodles and rinse in cold water to cool. Add them to a medium-size bowl and toss with a splash of sesame oil to keep them from sticking together. Set aside.

Prepare the chard, red cabbage, bell pepper, cucumber, carrot, and cilantro; set aside. In a blender, blend all the sauce ingredients (see next page) on high until smooth. Pour into a small serving bowl and set aside. Lay out all of your ingredients in assembly-line fashion (aka *mise en place*) and get ready to put the rolls together. Include a prepared protein source in your *mise en place* if desired. Pour warm water about ¼ inch deep onto a round plate or into a baking dish (large enough to accommodate the dimensions of a rice paper wrapper) and set aside another empty round plate. These will become your rice paper wrapper station. Now, you're ready to roll.

Start by dipping one rice paper wrapper into the warm water for about 20 seconds or until soft and pliable (replenish warm water as needed). Remove it and gently place it on the empty plate, unfolding any areas. In the center of the prepared wrapper, lay down a piece of rainbow chard vertically lengthwise and add 3 to 4 pieces of each prepared vegetable in a neat line in the middle of the leaf. Add a heaping line of oiled rice noodles on top of the vegetables, along with a healthy helping of cilantro leaves.

→

SAUCE

⅓ cup unsweetened creamy almond or peanut butter

2 inches fresh ginger (peel on OK if organic)

2 cloves garlic

¼ cup water

1 tablespoon plus 1 teaspoon soy sauce or gluten-free tamari

1 tablespoon rice wine vinegar

1 teaspoon honey or maple syrup

½ teaspoon red chili flakes or gochugaru

Starting at the bottom of the chard leaf (leaving the rice paper alone for now), roll it over the contents, tucking in any stray vegetables, finishing with the seam side down. Recenter the wrapped chard roll in the middle of the rice paper and fold the left and right edges of the rice paper in and over the chard roll. Next, gently wrap the bottom edge closest to you up and over the chard roll, continuing until fully wrapped and secured. I find that this process is easiest with wet hands. Set aside and repeat with the remaining rolls.

To prevent the completed rolls from sticking together, I rub a drop or two of sesame oil on the outside of each roll before stacking them together on a serving plate. Serve at room temperature or refrigerate for 20 minutes until cold and serve with the ginger almond butter dipping sauce. You can also wrap each roll in plastic wrap and refrigerate to enjoy at a later time. The rolls will store well in the refrigerator for 2 to 3 days before the rice paper wrapper will become chewy and start to dry out. The ginger almond butter sauce can be stored in a glass jar with an airtight lid and refrigerated up to 7 days.

The Simplest Tempeh Tacos
with Whole Wheat and Flax Tortillas

This is truly one of the simplest recipes and a great "gateway" tempeh recipe for beginners. Tempeh is fermented soybeans with many health benefits, including probiotics, plant-based protein, and fiber. Buy organic tempeh to ensure a quality product that's less processed and non-GMO. You can substitute ground chicken or turkey for the tempeh if you're looking for a meat-friendly version. MAKES 10-12 TACOS

DF | GF | V | Ve

2 tablespoons avocado oil

2 cups chopped white onion (about 1 large white onion)

1 teaspoon ground cumin

1 teaspoon ground coriander

½ teaspoon red chili flakes

¼ teaspoon cayenne

½ teaspoon sea salt

12 ounces organic soy tempeh, crumbled

2 cups (16 ounces) tomato salsa

1 cup thinly sliced red cabbage (about ¼ small head)

¼ cup chopped fresh cilantro

1 avocado, sliced

1 lime, cut into wedges

10–12 Whole Wheat and Flax Tortillas (recipe follows) or whole grain tortillas

Queso fresco, crumbled (optional)

Heat the oil in a large cast iron skillet or sauté pan over medium heat. Add the onion and sauté until translucent, about 5 to 7 minutes. Add the spices and salt, and sauté for an additional 30 seconds or until fragrant. Add the tempeh and salsa; sauté until warm and heated through (tempeh does not require cooking).

Remove from the heat and serve with warmed Whole Wheat and Flax Tortillas or any other tortillas. Top with some cabbage, cilantro, sliced avocado, and a squeeze of lime. Feel free to add cheese and any other beloved taco fixings.

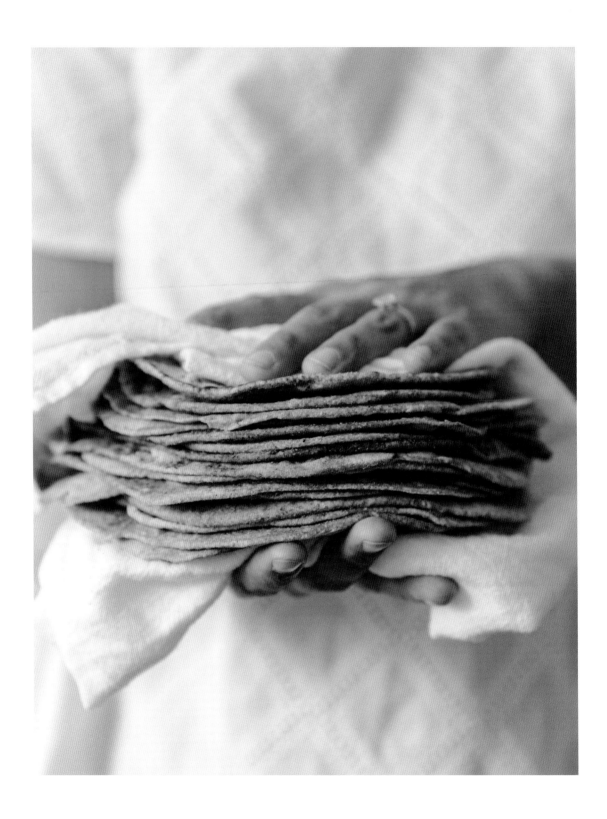

Whole Wheat and Flax Tortillas

Once you make your own tortillas, you'll wonder why it took you so long to ditch the store-bought variety. The combination of whole wheat flour and flaxseed meal in this recipe unites craveable carbs with amplified health benefits (think fiber, healthy fat, and B vitamins)—an obvious choice for your next Taco Tuesday! MAKES 16 TORTILLAS

DF | V | Ve | RT

2 cups whole wheat flour

¼ cup golden flaxseed meal (ground golden flaxseeds)

1 teaspoon sea salt

¼ cup olive oil

1 cup warm water

Whisk together the whole wheat flour, flaxseed meal, and salt in a large bowl. Add the olive oil and, with a clean pair of hands, mix it in until completely incorporated and the flour resembles coarse sand. Gradually add the warm water and mix with a fork until a loose ball forms. If your dough is too sticky, add more whole wheat flour. If your dough is too crumbly or scaly, add 1 tablespoon of warm water at a time.

Turn out the dough onto a floured surface; knead until smooth and slightly springy, about 1 to 2 minutes. Pinch off ping-pong-size balls and, with firm pressure between your palms, roll each into a smooth ball. You should have around 16 dough balls. Place them on a plate and cover with plastic wrap or a slightly damp dish towel and let rest at room temperature for 30 minutes.

Once the dough has rested, preheat a dry cast iron skillet on medium heat while preparing the tortillas. On a lightly floured surface, using a rolling pin (my preferred way) or tortilla press, roll out one tortilla at a time until fairly thin, circular(ish), and about 6 to 7 inches in diameter while keeping the remaining dough balls covered. Cook each tortilla for 45 to 60 seconds on each side, or until brown in spots and bubbling with small air pockets. The tortillas should be flexible and soft. If you overcook them, they will become brittle. Prepare the next tortilla while each is cooking. Remove from the heat and serve immediately for the best flavor and texture. Keep them warm by wrapping them in a clean dish towel or using a tortilla warmer.

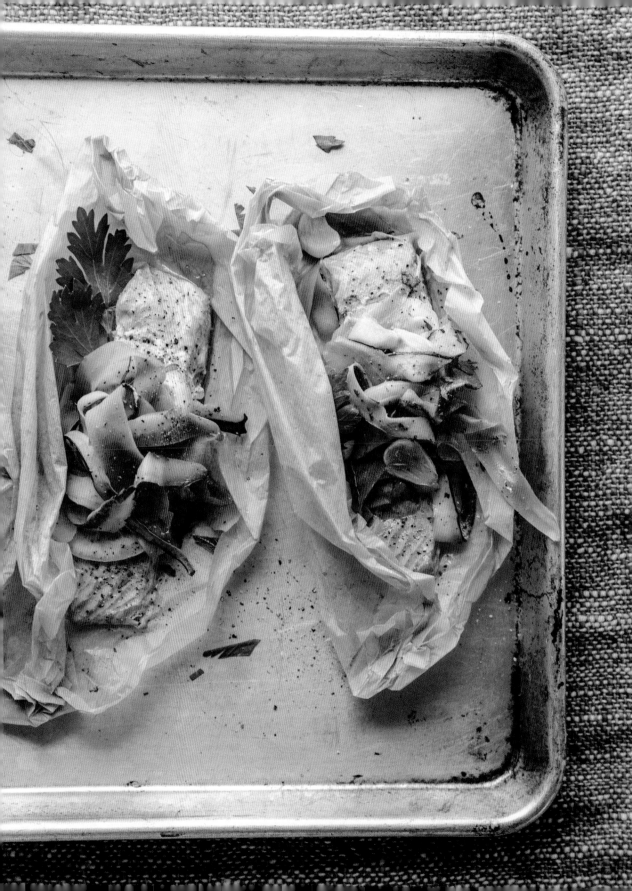

Salmon en Papillote
with Seasonal Vegetable Ribbons

In French cuisine, *en papillote* refers to cooking or steaming food in parchment or paper pockets. This simple technique is the perfect cooking method for more delicate proteins like fish and for maintaining the most nutrients. Four ounces of salmon contains well over the recommended Daily Value (DV) of vitamins B_{12} and D, and it's a great source of omega-3 fatty acids. SERVES 4

DF | GF

Four 4-ounce salmon fillets (skin on or off)

Sea salt and ground black pepper

1 small zucchini

2 large carrots

2 cloves garlic, peeled and thinly sliced crosswise

1 tablespoon olive oil

1 lemon, sliced paper-thin

Chopped flat-leaf parsley (garnish)

Prepare the parchment paper pockets. Cut four 18-inch-long pieces of parchment paper and fold each in half crosswise, creasing the paper at the fold. Using scissors, cut a semicircle on the folded parchment paper, using the creased side as the middle of the circle. Discard the pieces you cut off. When you open the folded paper, you should reveal a symmetrical circle. Complete four parchment circles and set aside.

Preheat oven to 425°F. Wash and thoroughly dry each salmon fillet with paper towels; salt and pepper all sides. Place on a dry plate and set aside.

Using a vegetable peeler, start at one end of the zucchini (keep the peel if it's organic) and peel long ribbons from the top to the bottom until you can't comfortably hold and peel any more. You should have about 1 cup of zucchini ribbons. Place in a medium-size mixing bowl. Do the same to the carrots, peeling long carrot ribbons for about 1 cup total. Add the carrots to the mixing bowl with the garlic and olive oil, and toss until well combined.

Prepare one salmon pocket at a time. Put a parchment circle (see note on page 160) on a baking sheet and place one fillet skin-side down (if skin on) on one half of the circle. Place 2 slices of lemon directly on top of the fillet. Top with a small handful (about ¼ cup) of the vegetable mixture. Fold the other half of the parchment circle over the salmon and vegetables and crimp the sides together along the rounded edge, folding tightly to completely seal the pocket closed while making sure to leave some air space in the center of the pocket. Repeat with the other fillets until you have four sealed salmon pockets arranged on one or two baking sheets.

→

Parchment paper works best for making the pockets, but foil is a good alternative when needed. You can substitute any type of fish in this recipe. Adjust the cooking time as needed, depending on the thickness of the fish. Other seasonal vegetable variations I like include asparagus ribbons and basil (spring), thinly sliced fennel and lemon (autumn), and thinly sliced blood orange and shallots (winter).

Place the baking sheet(s) in the oven and bake for 10 to 12 minutes until the fish is cooked through. Use less baking time for thinner pieces of fish and more for thicker pieces.

To serve, place one pocket on each dinner plate for diners to open (my preferred way). Alternatively you can unwrap all the pockets, remove the salmon and vegetables with a spatula, and serve them together on a platter. Garnish with parsley and season to taste with salt and pepper.

Flourless Chocolate Almond Butter Brownies

This flourless brownie recipe will satisfy almost any sweet tooth. It's chocolatey, gluten-free, dairy-free, refined sugar–free, and packed with healthy fats and more than 6 grams of protein per brownie. Also, almond butter helps to stabilize after-meal rises in blood sugar while providing beneficial antioxidants, so this really is a wholesome dessert. SERVES 9

DF | GF | V

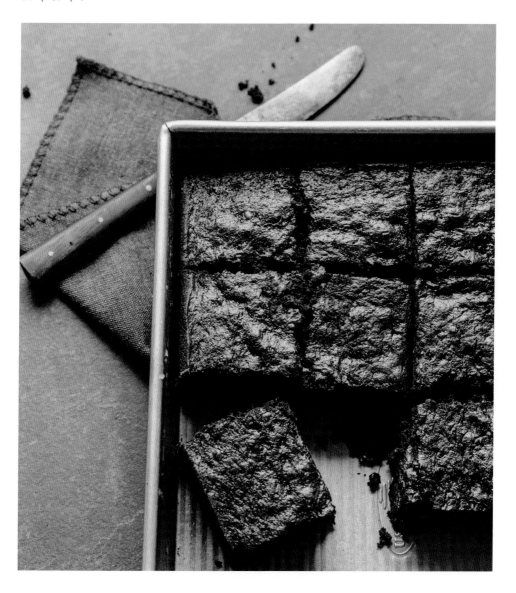

Coconut oil

1½ cups unsweetened creamy almond butter

2 eggs

¾ cup maple syrup

1 tablespoon vanilla extract

⅓ cup unsweetened cocoa powder, sifted

1 teaspoon baking soda

½ teaspoon sea salt

1 cup bittersweet chocolate chips

Preheat oven to 325°F. Oil an 8-inch square cake pan with coconut oil and set aside.

In a large mixing bowl with a fork or stand mixer with a paddle attachment, blend the almond butter, eggs, maple syrup, and vanilla together until smooth. In a separate small bowl, mix together the cocoa powder, baking soda, and salt; add to the wet mixture and blend until thoroughly combined. Fold in the chocolate chips.

Pour the brownie batter into the cake pan and use a spatula or the back of a spoon to smooth out the top. Bake for 35 to 40 minutes or until a toothpick inserted in the center comes out clean. Remove from the oven and let cool for at least 10 minutes before slicing and serving (if you can wait that long!), as the brownies will solidify and make cutting easier. Once they are completely cooled, store them in an airtight container at room temperature for up to 1 week.

Bittersweet chocolate is another name for dark chocolate used in baking. The package is typically labeled with a percentage of cacao which represents the cacao/sugar ratio. The higher the percentage of cacao, the more bitter the chocolate will be. I prefer bittersweet chocolate chips that are 60% to 70% cacao for this recipe for optimal sweetness and flavor.

Blueberry Acai and Coconut Ice Pops

These dairy-free, vegan ice pops are an effortlessly delightful summer dessert. Acai berries are native to South America and taste similar to red grapes or pomegranate seeds. They contain generous amounts of anthocyanin—a powerful compound that may help prevent cardiovascular disease and cancer and support cognitive function. Paired with blueberries, they make quite the impressive team!

You will need 6 to 8 ice pop molds (or small paper cups) and sticks for this recipe.

MAKES 6-8 ICE POPS

DF | GF | V | Ve | RT

One 13.5-ounce can unsweetened coconut cream or full-fat coconut milk

½ cup fresh or frozen blueberries

One 3-4-ounce frozen packet unsweetened acai purée

3 tablespoons honey or maple syrup

In a high-powered blender, blend all ingredients together until smooth and creamy, about 1 minute. You can blend for less time if you want visible pieces of fruit in the finished product; the flavor will be essentially the same.

Pour the coconut fruit purée into the individual ice pop molds, insert the sticks, and cover per the manufacturer's instructions. If you're using small paper cups, fill each cup with purée and cover with foil. Gently poke a hole in the foil with a popsicle stick and lower it into the cup. The foil will keep the stick standing upright.

Freeze the ice pops for at least 6 hours or until solidified. Remove individual ice pops from the freezer as needed and briefly run warm water over each mold to release the pop. Enjoy immediately. Store leftover ice pops in the freezer for up to 1 month.

> You can substitute almost any seasonal fruit in this recipe by using about 1 cup fresh or frozen fruit in place of the blueberries and acai. Some of my other favorite flavors include cantaloupe and cucumber, passion fruit (without the seeds) and pineapple, or raspberry and peach. Adjust the sweetener as needed.

8

AUTUMN

Autumn—the season of letting go. The leaves fall as a reminder for us to let go of what no longer serves us. Our external and internal climates begin to retreat, preparing us for cooler and crisper days ahead. We shift inward and reflect. We slow down and find value in rest.

Our appetite increases, our meals grow larger and less frequent, and our digestion slows. Starchy and stewed vegetables, hearty greens, whole grains, healthy fats, and animal proteins or hearty plant-based proteins serve us well this time of year. We relish the seasonal harvest of pumpkin, beets, cauliflower, apples, and cranberries to support and nourish us.

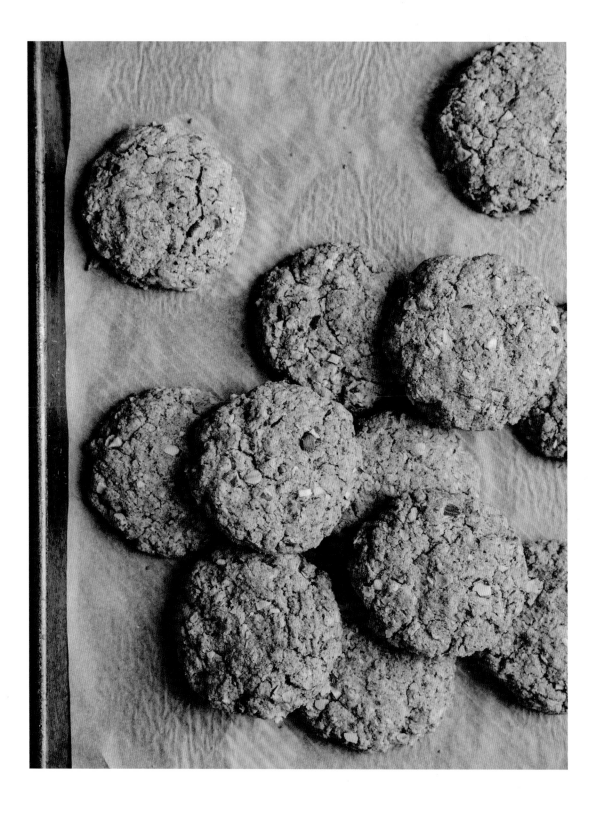

Roasted Banana and Almond Butter Breakfast Cookies

These breakfast cookies are a beloved go-to for my family and many of my patients. They're perfect for those busy bodies that often skip breakfast. Not only are they convenient and tasty (roasted bananas are the best!), but they also contain 7 grams of protein per cookie. That is something everyone can get behind. MAKES 1 DOZEN COOKIES

DF | GF | V | Ve

2 bananas, peeled

3 tablespoons maple syrup, divided

Pinch of ground cinnamon

1 cup quick-cooking rolled oats or quinoa flakes

2 cups superfine almond flour (natural or blanched)

½ teaspoon baking powder

½ teaspoon baking soda

¼ teaspoon sea salt

1 cup unsweetened creamy almond butter

2 tablespoons coconut oil, melted

1½ teaspoons vanilla extract

¼ cup finely chopped raw almonds

¼ cup finely chopped raw walnuts

Preheat oven to 400°F. Place whole bananas on a baking sheet lined with parchment paper. Drizzle 1 tablespoon of the maple syrup over the bananas and sprinkle with cinnamon. Roast in the oven for 15 minutes or until juices are golden brown. Remove from the oven and set aside to cool. Reduce oven temperature to 325°F.

Mix together the oats or quinoa flakes, almond flour, baking powder, baking soda, and salt in a large mixing bowl. In a separate large bowl, mash the cooled bananas with the back of a fork. Add the almond butter, coconut oil, 2 tablespoons maple syrup, and vanilla to the bananas; mix well. Using a spatula, add the dry ingredients to the wet ingredients and stir until combined (you don't have to worry about overmixing this dough since there's no wheat flour/gluten involved). At this point, your dough should have the consistency of sticky cookie dough. Finally, fold in the chopped nuts. I find that using clean hands works best at this stage.

Using a ¼-cup measure, scoop out the dough and roll it into balls with your hands. Place the balls on a parchment-lined baking sheet, 1 inch apart, and gently flatten into rounded disks. These cookies do not flatten or spread while cooking, so it's important that you shape them before baking. Make sure all the cookies are relatively the same size, so they bake evenly. Bake for 18 minutes or until the cookies are lightly golden brown on the bottom. Do not wait for the tops to turn golden brown or they will be too dry. Remove from the oven and let cool completely before enjoying with your favorite morning beverage.

Cinnamon Apple Overnight Oats
with Toasted Walnuts

This recipe reminds me of the flavors in apple pie. The rolled oats, chia seeds, and apple make this a great fiber-forward option to help you *break* your morning *fast* and satisfy your hunger. Alongside healthy fats and protein, these overnight oats are a good choice for anyone looking to maintain healthy blood glucose levels. Remember to use organic milk and yogurt whenever possible to ensure a quality breakfast with optimal nutrition. SERVES 8 (8-OUNCE SERVINGS) OR 4 (16-OUNCE SERVINGS)

DF | GF | V | Ve

½ cup raw walnuts

3 cups rolled oats

2 tablespoons chia seeds

1 teaspoon ground cinnamon

½ teaspoon ground ginger

¼ teaspoon ground nutmeg

3 cups whole milk or plant-based alternative

1 cup plain whole milk yogurt or plant-based alternative

¼ cup maple syrup

½ teaspoon vanilla extract

1½ cups finely chopped apples (about 2 small apples)

Preheat oven to 300°F. Spread the walnuts on a baking sheet and bake for 15 to 20 minutes or until they are fragrant and lightly toasted. Remove from the oven and set aside to cool. When cool enough to handle, chop the walnuts into small pieces. Set aside.

In a large mixing bowl, mix together the rolled oats, chia seeds, cinnamon, ginger, and nutmeg. In a medium-size bowl, whisk together the milk, yogurt, maple syrup, and vanilla; add to the dry ingredients, stirring thoroughly with a wooden spoon or spatula until well combined. At this point, your oat mixture should be wet and thick yet easily spoonable. Add more milk if needed. Finally, fold in the apples.

Set out either eight 8-ounce jars or four 16-ounce jars with lids. Spoon the oat mixture with apples into each jar, filling it at least three-quarters of the way or until the oats are evenly divided. Sprinkle toasted walnuts on top of each jar and screw on the lids.

Place the jars in the refrigerator overnight or for at least 8 hours. The longer you refrigerate them, the softer the oats become. When ready to eat, serve cold directly from the jar or gently heat the oats for 1½ to 2 minutes, making sure not to overheat them, which can make them gummy (if this happens, thin the warmed oat mixture with additional milk or yogurt).

Broccoli Salad
with Pickled Cranberries and Herb Yogurt Dressing

Broccoli is one of the most nutrient-dense vegetables out there. It's loaded with vitamin C, folate, vitamin K, and many other valuable nutrients. It's part of the cruciferous vegetable family that promotes natural detoxification and has been shown to decrease cancer risk and increase heart health. SERVES 8-10

GF | V

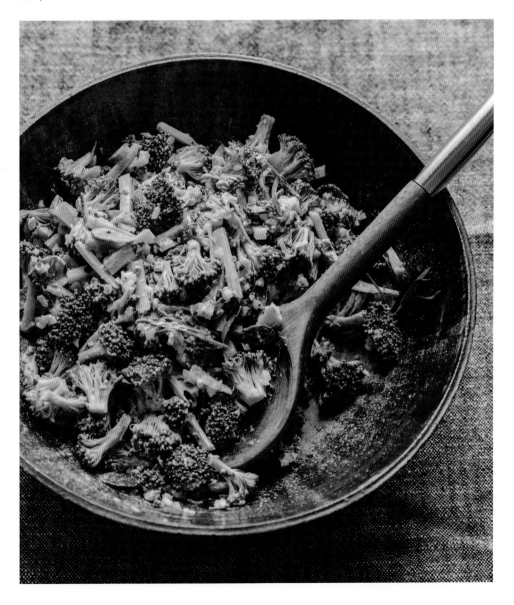

SALAD

½ cup dried cranberries (I prefer apple juice–sweetened)

¾ cup apple cider vinegar

6 cups broccoli florets (about 2 broccoli heads)

6 cups broccoli stalks, finely chopped or shredded (from 2 broccoli heads)

½ cup sliced almonds, toasted

¼ cup finely chopped red onion

DRESSING

1 cup plain whole-milk yogurt

1 tablespoon maple syrup

3 tablespoons finely chopped fresh tarragon (plus more for garnish)

1 tablespoon finely chopped fresh parsley (plus more for garnish)

⅓ cup blue cheese crumbles

1 teaspoon sea salt

¼ teaspoon ground black pepper

Start by quick-pickling the cranberries. Soak them in apple cider vinegar in a small bowl for at least 20 minutes, until they are plump and saturated (the longer the soak time, the better!). Drain and add to a large mixing bowl. You can forgo quick-pickling the cranberries if you'd like and just add dried cranberries directly to the bowl. Next, add the broccoli florets and stalks, almonds, and red onion. Mix together until combined.

In a medium bowl, mix together all dressing ingredients. Pour the dressing over the broccoli salad and mix together until the salad is evenly coated. Refrigerate for 20 to 30 minutes or until cool. Give the salad a quick stir and garnish with additional tarragon and parsley before serving.

Tangy Italian Cauliflower Salad

with Olives and Capers

Did you know that 1 cup of raw cauliflower contains almost 73 percent of the suggested amount of vitamin C needed per day (also known as the Daily Value)? Vitamin C is probably best known as an antioxidant, but it also helps us absorb iron, so make sure to eat your iron-rich foods with a little vitamin C. In this recipe, the cauliflower supplies the vitamin C, and the almonds and olives provide some iron. SERVES 8-10

DF | GF | V | Ve

1 medium cauliflower head

1 cup sliced almonds, toasted

½ cup black olives, pitted and chopped small (I prefer dry oil-cured black olives)

2 tablespoons finely diced red onion

2 tablespoons capers, drained

½ cup chopped flat-leaf parsley

¼ cup olive oil

2 tablespoons white wine vinegar

¼ teaspoon sea salt

Remove and discard the cauliflower leaves and the thickest part of the bottom stem; cut the head into 4 to 6 large pieces. Use a food processor with a 6-mm slicing disc or a mandoline set to the ¼-inch setting to slice the cauliflower into thin, bite-size pieces. A sharp knife and some patience work well too.

Place the sliced cauliflower, toasted almonds, olives, red onion, capers, and parsley in a large mixing bowl. In a small bowl, whisk together the oil, vinegar, and salt; pour over the cauliflower mixture and mix until well combined. Serve at room temperature, or refrigerate for 20 or more minutes or until chilled.

Roasted cauliflower works well as a substitute for raw cauliflower in this recipe. Cut one head of cauliflower into small florets and roast on a baking sheet at 400°F for about 20 minutes or until tender and lightly golden. Toss with the other ingredients and the dressing and serve warm or chilled.

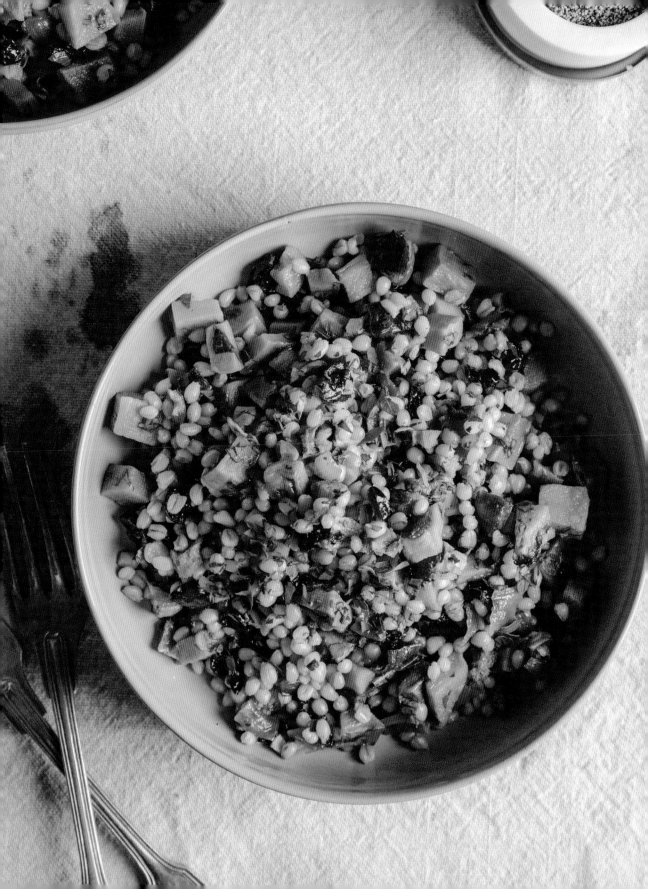

Wheat Berry Salad
with Butternut Squash and Maple Vinaigrette

Wheat berries are whole wheat grain kernels and a perfect example of a whole grain. You can easily substitute wheat berries in most rice or barley dishes to give them a chewy texture and nutty flavor. Wheat berries also deliver a healthy dose of fiber, protein, B vitamins, manganese, and magnesium. If you can't find wheat berries at your local market, you can substitute farro, which is another fantastic whole grain derived from a different species of wheat. SERVES 6-8

DF | V | Ve

- 1½ cups wheat berries, rinsed and drained
- ½ butternut squash, sliced lengthwise, seeded and peeled, cut into ½-inch cubes (about 3 cups)
- ½ medium red onion, finely chopped (about ½ cup)
- 1 teaspoon plus 2 tablespoons olive oil, divided
- 3 tablespoons apple cider vinegar
- 2 tablespoons maple syrup
- 1 teaspoon sea salt
- ½ cup dried cranberries (I prefer apple juice–sweetened)
- ¼ cup flat-leaf parsley, finely chopped

> If you're planning ahead, soak the wheat berries or farro in water for at least 8 hours or overnight. Drain and rinse before cooking.

Preheat oven to 400°F. Place the wheat berries in a medium-size saucepan and cover with at least 2 inches of water (about 6 cups). Bring to a boil over high heat, then reduce to low and cook the wheat berries, uncovered, for about 60 minutes; they should be tender but still slightly chewy or al dente. If you're using soaked grains, plan to reduce the cooking time even more. Once the grains reach the desired texture, remove from the heat and drain off any excess water. Set aside.

Place the squash on an unlined baking sheet and roast in the oven for 30 to 40 minutes or until fork tender. Remove from the oven and set aside to cool. Sauté the onions with 1 teaspoon of olive oil in a small frying pan on medium to high heat until translucent and tender, about 5 minutes. Set aside to cool.

In a large mixing bowl, whisk together the remaining 2 tablespoons of oil, vinegar, maple syrup, and salt. Add the wheat berries, squash, onions, and cranberries to the mixing bowl and combine. Allow the salad to sit for at least 20 minutes to give the wheat berries time to absorb some of the dressing. Season with additional salt to taste. Give the salad one more stir before garnishing with chopped parsley and serving at room temperature.

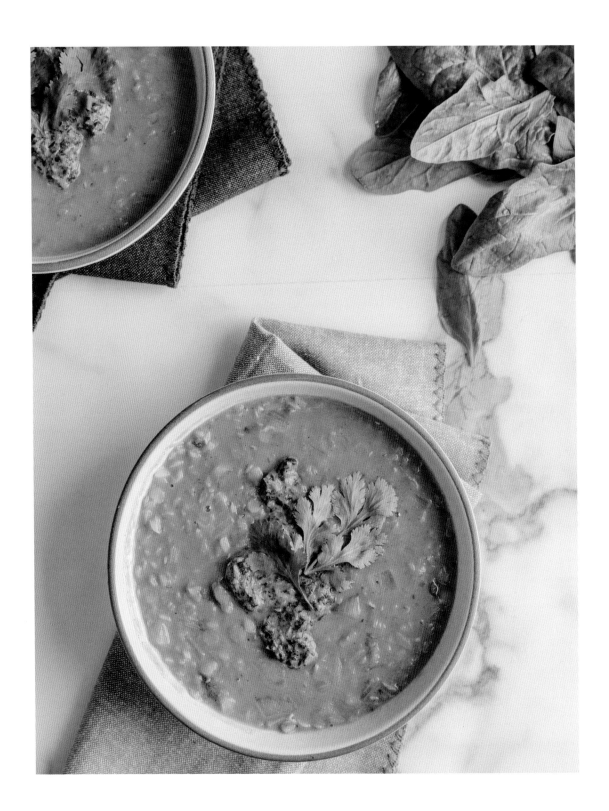

Coconut Curry Red Lentil Stew
with Cilantro Lime Chutney

This recipe is adapted from Angela Liddon's Glowing Spiced Lentil Soup from her popular plant-based food blog, *Oh She Glows*. Red lentils are a fantastic source of fiber making this hearty stew a heart-healthy go-to. With 90 percent of the Daily Value (DV) of folate and 37 percent of the DV of iron for every 1 cup of cooked lentils consumed, this recipe is a perfect choice for women looking to optimize their essential nutrient intake and promote reproductive health. SERVES 8–10

DF | GF | V | Ve

LENTIL STEW

1 tablespoon coconut oil or Ghee (page 101)

1 cup chopped yellow onion (about 1 medium onion)

3 garlic cloves, peeled and minced

1 tablespoon ground turmeric

1 teaspoon ground cumin

½ teaspoon ground black pepper

¼ teaspoon ground cardamom

¼–½ teaspoon cayenne

1 whole cinnamon stick

2 teaspoons sea salt

One 28-ounce can diced tomatoes with juices

Two 13.5-ounce cans unsweetened full-fat coconut milk

4 cups vegetable broth

1½ cups red lentils

1 large bunch spinach, destemmed and roughly chopped (about 3 cups)

Melt the coconut oil or ghee in a Dutch oven or stockpot over medium heat. Add the onion and sauté until tender and translucent. Add the garlic, turmeric, cumin, black pepper, cardamom, cayenne (½ teaspoon if you like it spicy), cinnamon stick, and salt; sauté for 30 seconds or until the spices bloom and become fragrant. Alternatively, substitute 1–2 tablespoons Golden Turmeric Paste (page 103) for the turmeric, cumin, black pepper, and cardamom.

Add the tomatoes and their juices, coconut milk, broth, and lentils to the Dutch oven, and stir until combined. Increase the heat to high and bring to a boil, then reduce the heat to low and let simmer uncovered for 15 to 20 minutes or until the lentils are tender and cooked through. Be mindful of the cinnamon stick in the stew and move aside or discard before serving.

Meanwhile, make the Cilantro Lime Chutney (see next page). In a small food processor or blender, blend the cilantro, scallions, lime juice, and sea salt until finely chopped but not fully puréed (I prefer mine a little chunky). With the food processor on, drizzle in the olive oil slowly and blend until the mixture has a pesto-like consistency. Pour into a smaller serving bowl or jar and season to taste with additional salt if needed. Set aside.

→

CILANTRO LIME CHUTNEY

1 bunch cilantro

4 scallions

Juice of 1 lime

¼ teaspoon sea salt

2 tablespoons olive oil

Add a small handful of chopped spinach to the bottom of every empty soup bowl used for serving. Ladle the stew into the bowl(s) on top of the spinach; the residual heat of the stew will soften the spinach. If you prefer, you can mix the spinach into the stew and cook it down for 1 to 2 minutes before ladling into bowls. Top each bowl with a spoonful of Cilantro Lime Chutney and serve warm.

To keep leftovers for more than a few days, freeze the stew in 1-quart glass jars with lids, leaving one to two inches of headspace. This will keep for 2 to 3 months.

Roasted Chicken Salad
with Grapes and Poppy Seed Yogurt Dressing

This recipe is simple, healthy, and delicious! Serve a large spoonful on a bed of massaged kale, stuff it inside a whole wheat pita, or eat it straight from the bowl. I recommend skinless white meat chicken in all of your chicken recipes if you need to reduce your dietary fat and cholesterol intake. I typically use a combination of skinless white and dark meat in my chicken recipes to boost the flavor. You can replace the chicken in this recipe with 4 cups of cooked or canned chickpeas (no need to bake) for a tasty vegetarian alternative. SERVES 8

GF

SALAD

2 boneless skinless chicken breasts (about 1½ pounds)

4 boneless skinless chicken thighs (about 1½ pounds)

¼ teaspoon salt

¼ teaspoon ground black pepper

1 cup chopped celery stalks (about 2 celery stalks)

1 cup halved red or green grapes

⅔ cup sliced almonds, toasted

2 tablespoons finely chopped red onion

1 tablespoon finely chopped fresh dill

1 tablespoon finely chopped flat-leaf parsley

DRESSING

¾ cup plain whole milk yogurt

1 tablespoon Dijon mustard

1½ teaspoons poppy seeds

¾ teaspoon sea salt

¼ teaspoon ground black pepper to taste

Preheat oven to 400°F. Place the chicken on a baking sheet and season both sides with salt and pepper. Bake for 15 to 20 minutes, or until chicken is cooked through but still moist. Remove from the oven and let cool slightly before handling. Cut the chicken into bite-size pieces or ½-inch cubes and add to a large mixing bowl. Add the rest of the salad ingredients to the same bowl and mix.

In a separate bowl, combine all dressing ingredients. Add the dressing to the salad and mix until fully combined. Cover the bowl and refrigerate for at least 20 minutes or until cool. Serve cold.

Mirin and Miso Glazed Cod

Cod is a relatively neutral-tasting white fish with many nutritional benefits. The protein and vitamin B12 content alone are quite impressive at about 20 grams of protein and about 60 percent of the Reference Daily Intake (RDI) of vitamin B12 per 6 ounces of fish. The combination of salty, sweet, and umami in this recipe makes this a well-balanced and flavorful choice. SERVES 6

DF | GF

Six 6-ounce skinless cod fillets

¼ cup mirin

2 tablespoons white miso paste

1 tablespoon toasted sesame oil

1 tablespoon honey

Turn the oven on to high broil. If using an oven with the heat source on top, place the oven rack 4 to 5 inches away from the top. If using an oven with the heat source on the bottom, use the heat/broil drawer below. Line a baking sheet with foil and set aside. Wash and thoroughly dry your cod; place it on the baking sheet, leaving room in between each fillet.

In a small bowl, whisk together the mirin, miso paste, oil, and honey. Liberally brush the top and sides of each fillet with the glaze and broil for 3 minutes. Remove from the oven and flip the fillets before brushing with the remaining glaze. Broil for another 3 to 5 minutes until cooked through and golden on top. Cooking time will vary depending on the thickness of each fillet. Thinner pieces closer to the tail end of the fish will need less broiling time. Remove from the oven and serve hot.

> Mirin is a sweet Japanese cooking wine made from rice. You can easily find it online and at most grocery stores in the international foods section. If necessary, you can substitute white wine or rice vinegar, but you'll want to increase the honey by about 1 tablespoon.

Skillet Roasted Lemon Chicken
with Green Olives and Garlic

This dish is a delicious ode to the Mediterranean. The olives are an excellent source of monounsaturated (healthy) fats, anti-inflammatory phytonutrients, and antioxidants. An interesting fact: crushing, chopping, or slicing garlic releases an enzyme called alliinase, which is responsible for the majority of garlic's health benefits, so always process your garlic before using it in a recipe. SERVES 4–6

DF | GF

1 pound whole baby potatoes

Sea salt

4 skin-on, bone-in whole chicken legs (separate skin-on thighs and drumsticks are OK)

Ground black pepper

2 tablespoons ghee

12 whole Castelvetrano or green olives, pitted

1 lemon (½ sliced paper-thin into 6–8 slices and ½ left whole)

8 whole garlic cloves, peeled and halved crosswise

1 tablespoon white wine vinegar

Preheat oven to 500°F. Place the potatoes in a large saucepan and cover with water by at least 2 inches; season generously with salt. Bring to a boil over high heat and cook until fork tender, anywhere from 8 to 12 minutes. Remove from the heat, drain, and let cool. When cool enough to handle, cut each potato in half crosswise and set aside.

Heat a large cast iron pan over medium to high heat. Thoroughly dry each chicken leg with a paper towel and liberally season both sides with salt and pepper. Add the ghee to the preheated pan and place the chicken in, skin-side down; cook until the skin browns, about 5 minutes. Turn the chicken over, skin-side up, and add the potatoes, olives, lemon slices, and garlic. Sprinkle the vinegar evenly over the potatoes, avoiding the chicken if possible (this will keep the chicken crispy).

Transfer your pan with the chicken to the oven and cook for 20 minutes until the chicken is cooked through and the skin is crispy. The potatoes, olives, lemon, and garlic should brown slightly and also become crisp. Remove from the oven and let the chicken rest for 10 to 15 minutes before serving directly from the pan. Season to taste with additional salt and pepper and/or a squeeze of lemon.

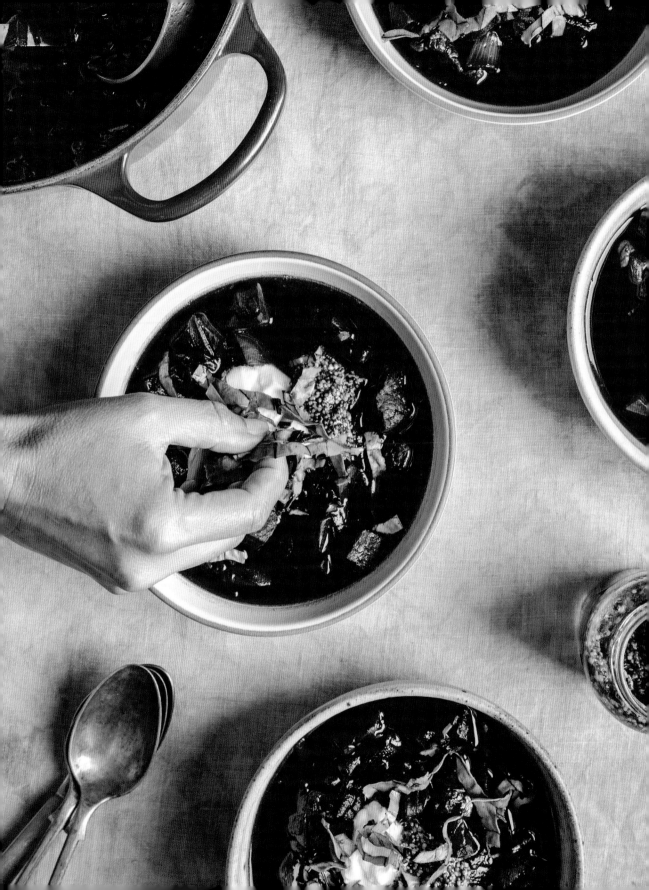

Beef and Beet Borscht
with Fresh Beet Greens

This recipe is inspired by one of my favorite chefs, Bonnie Morales, from the restaurant Kachka in Portland, Oregon. This colorful soup makes for an incredibly nourishing meal, especially for new mamas in the postpartum period. It provides protein, collagen, fiber, and electrolytes, as well as beneficial blood-building iron from the beets, beet greens, and beef. Also, there are probiotics from the yogurt! SERVES 6-8

GF | RT

2 pounds boneless beef short ribs or chuck roast (fat trimmed off), cut into 1-inch cubes

Sea salt and ground black pepper

1 tablespoon unsalted butter

6 red beets with greens attached

1 cup chopped yellow onion (about 1 medium yellow onion)

1 cup shredded carrots (about 2 large carrots)

2½ quarts low-sodium beef stock

Plain whole milk yogurt (garnish)

Whole grain mustard (garnish)

Thoroughly heat a Dutch oven or stockpot over medium to high heat. Liberally season the beef with salt and pepper while melting the butter. Using metal tongs, add the beef in batches, browning on all sides; allow about 5 minutes per batch, adding more butter if needed. Remove the beef and place on a plate lined with a paper towel; set aside. Turn off the heat and reserve the cooking oils left in the Dutch oven or pot.

Next, process the beets (peeling first if they are nonorganic). Reserve the greens but remove and discard the stems. Shred 3 beets and cut the remaining 3 into 1-inch cubes. Cut the beet greens into ¼-inch ribbons and set aside. Return your Dutch oven or pot to the stove and bring back to medium heat; add the shredded beets (not the cubes), onion, carrots, and 1 teaspoon salt. Sauté for 10 minutes or until the vegetables soften and the onions become translucent. Remove from the pot with a slotted spoon and set aside. Add the beet cubes and beef stock to the pot and bring to a boil. Reduce the heat, add the browned beef, and simmer covered for 1 to 1½ hours, or until the beef is tender. Return the onion, carrots, and shredded beets to the borscht and simmer for an additional 5 to 10 minutes. Season to taste with salt and pepper.

Prepare your soup bowls by adding a small handful of beet greens to the bottom of each bowl; ladle the borscht over the greens. The hot borscht will tenderize the greens. Top each bowl with a spoonful of yogurt and mustard. Serve hot.

If you are looking to keep the soup for more than a few days, it freezes well—store in an airtight container, such as a 1- quart glass jar with a lid, with 1 to 2 inches of headspace, for 2 to 3 months.

Chocolate Tofu Mousse
with Coconut Whip

This light and creamy chocolate mousse doesn't feel like a compromise or substitute for those looking for a vegan, dairy-free, refined sugar–free dessert. It's rich and chocolatey and has the added benefits of plant-based protein, calcium, and omega-3 fatty acids from the tofu. Make sure to use unsweetened cocoa powder, whenever possible, to minimize added sugar and maintain the highest nutritional value with the least amount of processing. Antioxidant-rich cacao nibs are a bonus! SERVES 4-6

DF | GF | V | Ve | RT

CHOCOLATE MOUSSE

12–14 ounces silken tofu

⅓ cup unsweetened coconut cream or full-fat coconut milk (solids only), nonrefrigerated

¼ cup maple syrup

3 tablespoons unsweetened cocoa powder

1½ teaspoons vanilla extract

COCONUT WHIP

One 13.5-ounce can unsweetened coconut cream or full-fat coconut milk, refrigerated for at least 8 hours or overnight

3 tablespoons maple syrup

1 teaspoon vanilla extract

OPTIONAL TOPPINGS

¼ cup large coconut flakes

Raw cacao nibs

Process all mousse ingredients together in a blender on high until smooth, about 45 to 60 seconds. Divide the mousse equally into ramekins or small glass jars; refrigerate uncovered for at least 2 hours. Ideally, you should let it set for at least 24 hours. The mousse will keep in the refrigerator for up to 3 days before it begins to separate.

Remove the can of coconut cream or milk from the refrigerator without shaking the can. Gently turn the can upside down before opening and discard the liquid on top. You should be left with only the coconut fat solids. Add the solids with all of the other coconut whip ingredients to an electric stand mixer fitted with the whisk attachment or to a large bowl with a handheld electric mixer. Beat on high speed for 2 to 3 minutes or until the mixture becomes light and fluffy and resembles traditional whipped cream. Adjust the sweetness to taste with additional maple syrup. Use immediately or store in an airtight container for up to 1 week (whisk to reconstitute if necessary).

Once the mousse is set and chilled, remove individual servings from the refrigerator as needed and add a large spoonful of coconut whip to each. You can also add optional toppings. Toast the coconut flakes in a small, dry sauté pan over medium heat for 2 to 3 minutes, stirring constantly until the edges are golden brown. Remove from the heat immediately and cool on a small plate. Additionally, you can use raw cacao nibs. Sprinkle topping(s) over the coconut whip and enjoy!

Mini Whole Wheat Apple Galettes
with Salted Honey

The smell of baked apples and cinnamon immediately transports me to autumn in the Pacific Northwest. Mmm . . . can you smell it? As research on the microbiome continues to develop, we are learning more about probiotics and what they "eat" or need to survive in the lower digestive tract. One fantastic source of *prebiotics*, or "food" for probiotics, comes from the pectin that naturally exists in apples. MAKES 4 MINI GALETTES

V | RT

CRUST

1½ cups whole wheat pastry flour

½ teaspoon sea salt

6 tablespoons cold unsalted butter, cut into ½-inch cubes

⅓–½ cup ice water

FILLING AND TOPPING

2 large or 3 small Granny Smith apples, cored, quartered, and sliced thin

Zest and juice of 1 small orange

Zest of 1 lemon

3 tablespoons maple syrup

1 teaspoon ground cinnamon

¼ teaspoon ground cardamom

¼ teaspoon ground nutmeg

1 egg

Honey

Large-flake sea salt or Maldon sea salt

In a large bowl, whisk together the flour and salt. Use clean hands to add the cold butter, breaking it apart with your fingers until the flour mixture resembles coarse crumbs. It's OK if there are a few large, buttery chunks remaining—these will become those flaky layers we love so much. Drizzle ice water in slowly, 1 tablespoon at a time, mixing with a wooden spoon just until a rough, shaggy ball forms. Your dough should barely stick together when squeezed.

Trying not to overhandle the dough, gently gather it and turn it out onto a lightly floured surface. Fold it over itself a couple of times (2 to 3 times is sufficient), bringing it together into one solid piece. Cut the dough into four even pieces and pat each piece into a small, flat disk. Tightly wrap each disk in plastic wrap and refrigerate for at least 1 hour, or up to 48 hours. You can also freeze the disks for 3 months; just thaw them in the refrigerator for 24 hours before using.

Meanwhile, preheat oven to 375°F. Make your apple filling by adding the apples, orange zest and juice, lemon zest, maple syrup, and spices to a large bowl; mix well.

Line a baking sheet with parchment paper and set aside. Remove your dough disks from the refrigerator and place one on a lightly floured surface. You may need to give the dough a minute or two to warm up slightly to make it easier to roll out. Using a lightly floured rolling pin, roll the dough into a ¼-inch-thick circle, turning and flipping regularly to keep it from sticking to your surface. (In my opinion, rough-edged asymmetrical "circles" make for better, more rustic-looking galettes.) Loosely cover the disk with plastic wrap and repeat for all the galette rounds.

→

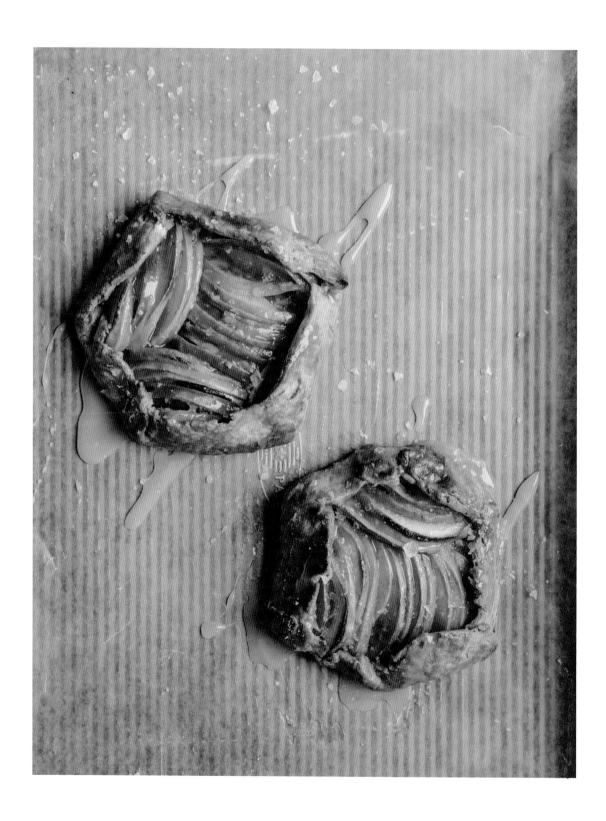

You can make 1 large galette instead of 4 small ones, if you prefer. Follow the recipe as shown, but increase the baking time to 45 to 55 minutes total.

Transfer each disk to the parchment-lined baking sheet. Fill with overlapping slices of apples in a single layer, tightly fanned or shingled across the pastry to leave a 1-inch border. Fold the dough border up and over the apples to create a crust. Brush the crust with an egg wash (whisked egg in a small bowl with a splash of water). Pour any remaining juices from the apple mixture evenly over the apple filling, but not on the crusts.

Bake for 30 to 40 minutes or until crust is golden brown, the juices are bubbling, and the apples are tender. Remove from the oven and let cool for 10 minutes. Drizzle each galette with a small spoonful of honey in a zigzag pattern—the sweetness of this dessert is dictated by the honey drizzle, so feel free to use more or less honey to match your taste. Finish with a healthy pinch of large-flake or Maldon sea salt. Enjoy the galettes warm or at room temperature.

9

WINTER

In the winter, we turn inward. We quietly contemplate
and surrender. As the plants and animals lie dormant
and hibernate, so should we. We are grateful for the
time spent preparing for these slow, calm days and
find our restraint useful and subtly energizing.

Our appetite grows heavier as our digestion slows.
Our meals are fewer but deeply nourishing. Starchy
and cooked vegetables, hearty grains, healthy fats,
and animal or hearty plant-based proteins support
and ground us. We're grateful for the sweet potatoes,
brussel sprouts, oranges, and kale this season affords.

Homemade Whole Wheat Toaster Waffles

These whole wheat waffles are crispy and light and have a delicious yeasted flavor—think homemade bread. I double the recipe whenever I make these and store the surplus in an airtight container or bag in my freezer for a quick and easy toaster waffle breakfast another day. Read more about batch cooking on page 116. Give it a try! MAKES 12–15 WAFFLES

V | RT

WAFFLES

½ cup warm water

2 teaspoons active dry yeast

2 tablespoons unsalted butter, melted

1½ cups whole milk, room temperature

2 cups whole wheat flour

½ teaspoon sea salt

3–4 tablespoons maple syrup

2 eggs

1 tablespoon vanilla extract

¼ teaspoon baking soda

OPTIONAL TOPPINGS

Butter and maple syrup

Almond butter and roasted bananas

Vanilla yogurt and fresh seasonal fruit

Nut butter and fruit jam

Smoked salmon and avocado

Mix together the water and yeast in a large mixing bowl; proof for 10 or more minutes, or until foaming. If your yeast doesn't foam, try a new batch. Add the butter, milk, flour, and salt to the yeast mixture and whisk together until smooth. Whisk in 3 tablespoons of maple syrup if you want a more savory waffle and 4 tablespoons if you like your waffles slightly sweeter. Your batter should be as thick as traditional waffle batter at this stage.

Cover the bowl loosely with plastic wrap or a damp towel and place in the oven (with the light on and the heat off) near the oven light. The light alone creates the perfect amount of heat. Let the batter rise in the oven for 60 minutes or until it doubles in size. Keep in mind the yeast flavor (sour, tangy) will get stronger the longer you let it rise. I find that 60 minutes is sufficient.

Remove the batter from the oven and preheat the oven to 200°F if you plan to eat the waffles immediately. Turn on your waffle iron and bring up to temperature (temperature varies depending on the iron). Whisk together the eggs, vanilla, and baking soda in a small mixing bowl and add to the batter, mixing gently until incorporated. I like to use a rubber spatula for this. It's OK if you deflate your batter slightly. Once all ingredients are combined, use a scoop to portion out batter into your waffle iron. The amount will depend on the size of your iron. I have a small vintage waffle iron, so I use a ¼-cup scoop and cook each waffle for 4½ to 5 minutes. Cook each waffle until crispy and golden brown on both sides. As you remove the hot waffles from the iron, place them directly on the rack in the preheated oven to keep warm and crispy until serving. When ready to eat, remove individual servings and top each waffle with your favorite toppings.

If you're batch cooking (see page 116) waffles for the freezer to eat at a later time, you can remove fresh waffles from the iron and cool to room temperature on a rack. Put the cooled waffles in a freezer bag or airtight container and label with today's date. If you put hot or warm waffles in a container or bag, they will get soggy. Keep the waffles in your freezer for up to 1 month. When you're ready to eat them, pop the frozen waffle(s) in the toaster or toaster oven and reheat for 2 to 3 minutes.

Chocolate and Chai Spiced Granola

This recipe combines two things I absolutely adore: dark chocolate and chai! Multiple whole grains and nuts make this a wonderful, nutrient-dense choice that I eat by the handful as a snack and as a topping on homemade yogurt or smoothie bowls. It also makes for a fun seasonal gift during the holidays, especially when presented in beautiful vintage glass jars.

MAKES ABOUT 6 CUPS

DF | GF | V | Ve

1¼ cups rolled oats

½ cup raw buckwheat groats

½ cup raw hazelnuts

½ cup quinoa flakes

½ cup large coconut flakes

¼ cup raw pecans, roughly chopped

¼ cup raw walnuts, roughly chopped

3 tablespoons unsweetened cocoa powder

1 teaspoon ground cardamom

1 teaspoon ground cinnamon

1 teaspoon ground ginger

½ teaspoon ground nutmeg

¼ teaspoon sea salt

¼ cup honey or maple syrup

3 tablespoons coconut oil

2 teaspoons vanilla extract

One 3-ounce bar 60%–70% cacao dark chocolate, finely chopped (about ½ cup)

Preheat oven to 325°F, arranging the rack in the center of the oven. In a large mixing bowl, combine the oats, groats, hazelnuts, quinoa flakes, coconut, pecans, and walnuts. In a smaller bowl, whisk together the cocoa powder and spices, including the salt; add to the large mixing bowl with the grain and nut mixture. Stir well until combined. Set aside.

Heat the honey or maple syrup and coconut oil in a small saucepan over low to medium heat until liquified, about 2 minutes. Do not boil. Remove from the heat and stir in the vanilla extract. Add the wet ingredients to the dry ingredients in the large bowl, and with a rubber spatula or wooden spoon, mix until thoroughly combined.

Spread the granola mixture evenly on a metal baking sheet and bake for 10 minutes. Remove from the oven, stir, and spread evenly over the baking sheet again. Bake for an additional 10 minutes. Remove from the oven and let cool for 5 minutes before transferring to a second room-temperature baking sheet. Add the chocolate pieces and stir well (I use clean hands). The residual heat of the granola will melt the chocolate slightly, incorporating it into the mixture while leaving some chocolate chunks. Let cool completely on the baking sheet for at least 20 to 30 minutes before enjoying, or you can put the baking sheet in the refrigerator to speed up the process. Store granola in a glass jar or container.

Buckwheat Breakfast Porridge
with Cranberry Chia Compote

This is a great alternative to traditional oatmeal, which can get a little boring, or most breakfast cereals that lack nutrition. The buckwheat and quinoa provide heart-healthy nutrients that also help you balance blood sugar, lower cholesterol and blood pressure, and may even prevent some forms of cancer. Be sure to choose dark red or even purple cranberries for the compote, versus lighter red or white ones, to ensure the highest amount of anthocyanin (disease-fighting compounds). SERVES 2-4

DF | GF | V | Ve | RT

PORRIDGE

½ cup raw buckwheat groats

½ cup tricolor quinoa

2 cups water

> If you're planning ahead, soak the buckwheat and quinoa together in water for at least 8 hours or overnight. Drain and rinse before cooking.

COMPOTE

10–12 ounces fresh or frozen cranberries

Zest and juice of 1 medium orange

2 inches fresh ginger, cut into 4 pieces

¼ cup maple syrup

2 tablespoons chia seeds

Add the buckwheat, quinoa, and water to a small saucepan and bring to a boil over high heat. Reduce the heat to a simmer and cover, cooking the grains until light and fluffy, about 20 minutes. If you're using soaked grains, reduce the cooking time. The grains should absorb all of the water once they're done cooking, but always taste-test for the optimal texture. This will yield about 3 to 3½ cups of cooked grains.

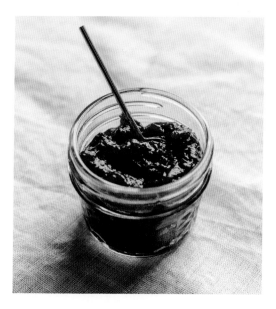

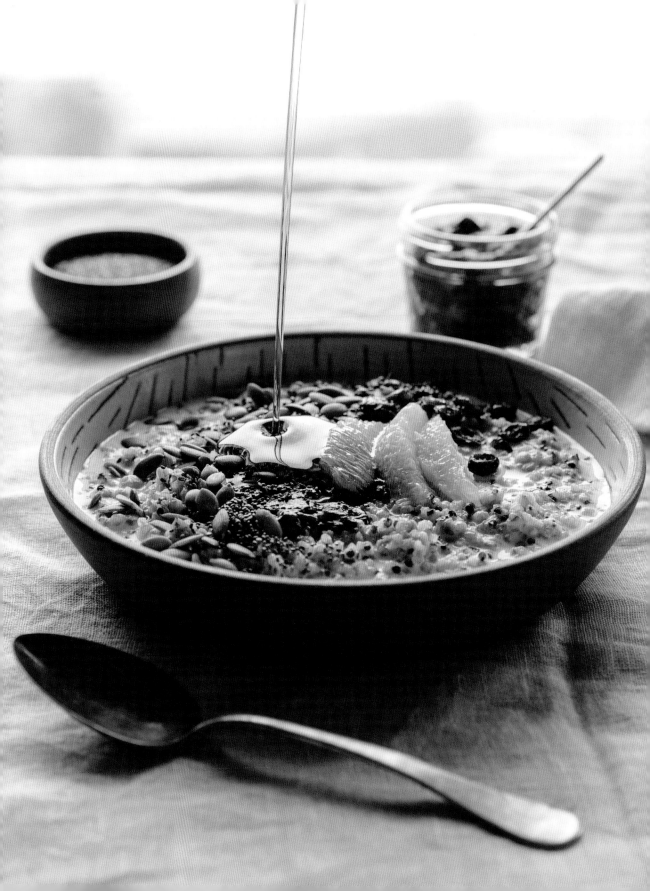

Milk

Maple syrup

Raw pumpkin seeds

Dried cranberries

Chia seeds

Segmented oranges

While the grains are cooking, make the compote. Put all ingredients, except the chia seeds, in a small saucepan over low to medium heat, stirring occasionally, until the cranberries burst open and break down and the sauce thickens, about 15 to 20 minutes. Toward the end, I use a wooden spoon to mash the remaining cranberries open and minimize any larger chunks.

Remove the compote from the heat and discard the ginger pieces. Add the chia seeds to the saucepan and stir until evenly incorporated. Let it cool slightly and allow time for the chia seeds to thicken the compote. Let the compote cool to room temperature before spooning into an 8-ounce glass container or jar with a lid and storing in the refrigerator for up to 1 week.

Spoon individual servings of porridge into bowls and top each with compote and the suggested toppings. Feel free to substitute your favorite toppings. Serve warm.

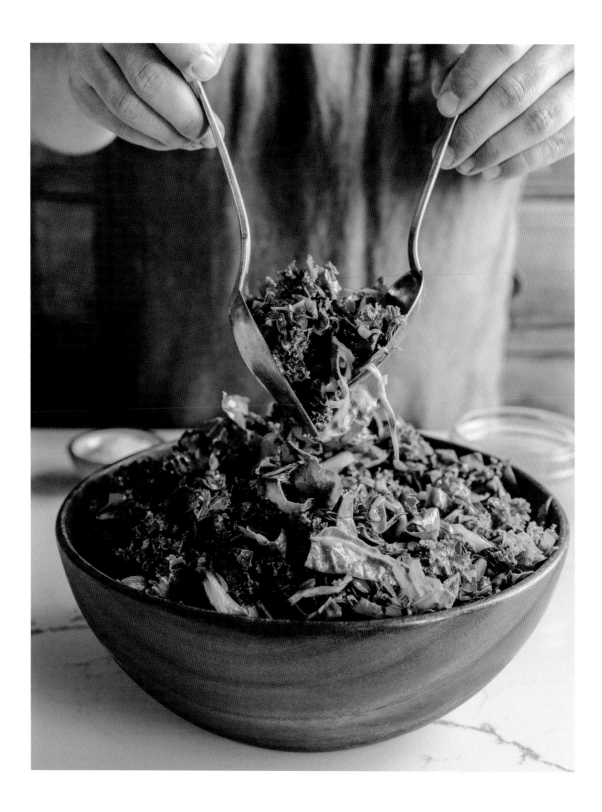

Curly Kale and Wild Rice Salad
with Sweet Fennel and Garlic Vinaigrette

This recipe is inspired by the Puget Consumers Co-op's (PCC's) Emerald City Salad. It's a fantastic green salad that makes for a fabulous entrée or side dish. It keeps well in the refrigerator due to the hearty greens and whole grains and actually gets better over time. Remember, to preserve the most nutrients in the garlic used for the vinaigrette, always use fresh garlic versus peeled, prepackaged, powder, or paste. SERVES 8-10

DF | GF | V | Ve

SALAD

1 cup wild rice (I prefer black), rinsed and drained

3 cups water

1 fennel bulb with stalks, trimmed and cut in ¼-inch-thick slices, fronds reserved

2 tablespoons olive oil, divided

1 teaspoon maple syrup

¼ teaspoon sea salt

1 bunch curly kale, stalks removed and discarded, leaves thinly sliced

½ bunch rainbow chard, stalks removed and finely chopped, leaves thinly sliced

¼ cup finely chopped flat-leaf parsley

DRESSING

1 whole garlic bulb

½ cup olive oil

Juice of 2 lemons (about 6 tablespoons)

½ teaspoon sea salt

> If you're planning ahead, soak the wild rice in water for at least 8 hours or overnight. Drain and rinse before cooking.

Preheat oven to 400°F. Combine the wild rice and water in a small saucepan over high heat. Bring to a boil, then reduce the heat to a simmer and cover; cook the rice for about 45 to 50 minutes. The rice should absorb all the water once it's done cooking, but always taste-test for the optimal texture. If you're using soaked rice, reduce the cooking time. Remove from the heat and carefully scoop the hot rice onto a baking sheet, spreading evenly, to cool. Set aside. This will yield about 3½ cups of cooked rice.

While the rice is cooking, start the salad dressing. Slice the top off the garlic, exposing the tops of the cloves, and place it in a small piece of aluminum foil. Drizzle with a ½ teaspoon olive oil and wrap tightly. Place the foiled-wrapped garlic directly on the oven rack and roast for 45 to 50 minutes or until each clove is soft, almost creamy, and easy to push out with your fingers. Remove from the oven and set aside.

Next, line a baking sheet with parchment paper and set aside. Toss the sliced fennel bulb and stalks in a large bowl with 1 tablespoon of the olive oil, the maple syrup, and the salt. Spread the fennel evenly on a baking sheet and roast for 20 minutes, or until softened and slightly browned or caramelized. Remove from the oven and set aside to cool.

→

Add the kale, 1 tablespoon olive oil, and a pinch of salt to a large bowl; massage with clean hands for 2 to 3 minutes until the kale softens and reduces in size by about a third. Massaging your kale will make it easier to chew and help with digestion. Add the chard (stalks and leaves), parsley, cooked and cooled rice, and cooled fennel to the bowl; toss together until combined.

Process all the dressing ingredients, including the roasted garlic, in a blender on high for 30 seconds or until fully emulsified. Pour over the salad and toss until all ingredients are evenly coated. Refrigerate for at least 20 minutes or until cool and ready to serve. Garnish with fennel fronds.

Spicy Three Bean Chili

This hearty chili is great served fresh or frozen for another time. Beans, especially pinto beans, are an exceptional source of folate. Folate supports healthy nervous system function, heart health, red blood cell production, and reproductive health in women. If using dried beans, remember to soak them in water for at least 12 hours or overnight before cooking to reduce the cooking time and increase digestibility! SERVES 8-10

DF | GF | V | Ve

¾ cup dried (or one
   15-ounce can) pinto beans

¾ cup dried (or one
   15-ounce can) kidney beans

¾ cup dried (or one
   15-ounce can) black beans

8 cups water

1 tablespoon olive oil

1 medium yellow onion,
   chopped (about 1 cup)

1 green bell pepper, chopped
   (about 1 cup)

2 poblano peppers, seeds
   removed, chopped (about
   1 cup)

2 jalapeño peppers, seeds
   removed and reserved
   (optional), diced (about
   ⅓ cup)

2 teaspoons sea salt

2 cloves garlic, peeled and diced

1 teaspoon chili powder

1 teaspoon dried oregano

½ teaspoon cumin

½ teaspoon cayenne

Two 14- to 15-ounce cans diced
   tomatoes

One 14- to 15-ounce can
   tomato sauce

3 cups vegetable stock

1 lime, cut into wedges

Plain whole milk yogurt or
   plant-based alternative
   (optional)

If using dried beans, combine all the beans in a large sauce-pan with 8 cups water; add more water if necessary to cover the beans completely. Cook over high heat until boiling, then reduce the heat to simmer and cover. Cook the beans for 1 to 1½ hours or until tender. Soaking the beans ahead of time should help the different beans cook at the same rate. If one type of bean takes longer to cook, that's fine; the others can tolerate the difference. Also note, the older your dried beans, the longer they will take to cook. Drain the cooked beans and set aside. You can skip this step and save substantial time by substituting canned beans (drained and rinsed).

Heat the oil in a large stockpot over medium to high heat; add the onion, all peppers (and the jalapeño pith and seeds if you like it spicy), and the salt. Sauté for 5 to 7 minutes or until the onions are translucent. Add the garlic and spices, and cook for an additional 30 seconds. Add the diced tomatoes, tomato sauce, and vegetable stock; bring to a boil. Reduce the heat to low, add the cooked or canned beans, and simmer for an additional 20 minutes or until the beans are heated through. If you like a thicker chili, you can simmer it for longer to reduce the liquid. Season to taste. Garnish with a squeeze of lime and a spoonful of yogurt (optional).

If you'd like to keep leftovers longer than a couple of days, store the chili in the freezer, with one to two inches of head-space in the container, for 2 to 3 months.

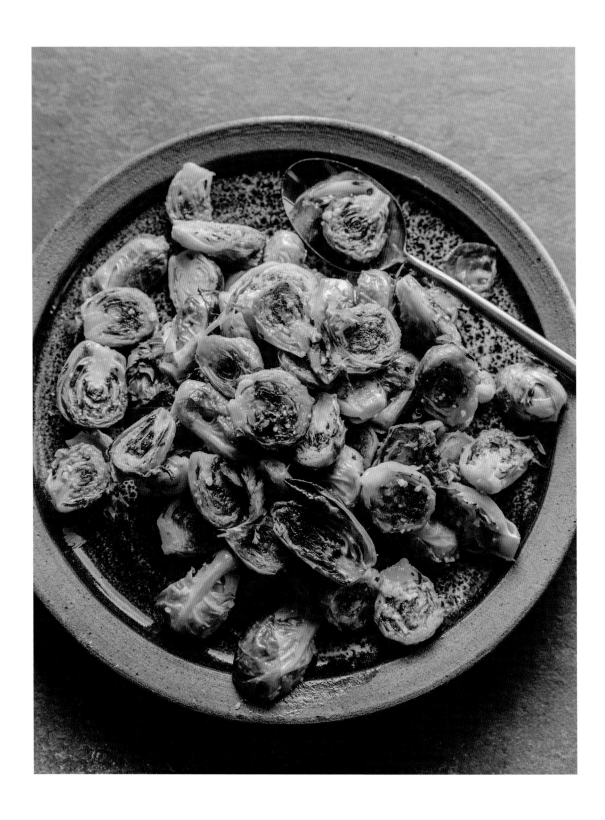

Roasted Brussel Sprouts
with Honey Miso Glaze and Cilantro

Brussel sprouts are one of the most well-studied vegetables in relation to cancer prevention. They are incredibly beneficial for the body's natural detoxification system, aid antioxidant function, and provide anti-inflammatory properties. They're also loaded with vitamins C and K and folate. Seconds, please! SERVES 4

DF | GF

1½ pounds brussel sprouts, ends trimmed and halved

1 tablespoon toasted sesame oil

1 teaspoon fish sauce

2 tablespoons white miso paste

1 tablespoon plus 1 teaspoon honey

1 tablespoon rice wine vinegar

2 tablespoons chopped fresh cilantro

Preheat oven to 425°F. Place the brussel sprouts in a large bowl and toss with the sesame oil to coat. Spread the brussel sprouts in a single layer on a baking sheet, cut sides down, and roast for 15 to 20 minutes until browned and tender.

While the sprouts are roasting, add the remaining ingredients, except for the cilantro, to the same large mixing bowl and whisk until well combined. When the sprouts are done, remove from the oven and place on a serving plate. Drizzle with the glaze and garnish with cilantro. Serve warm.

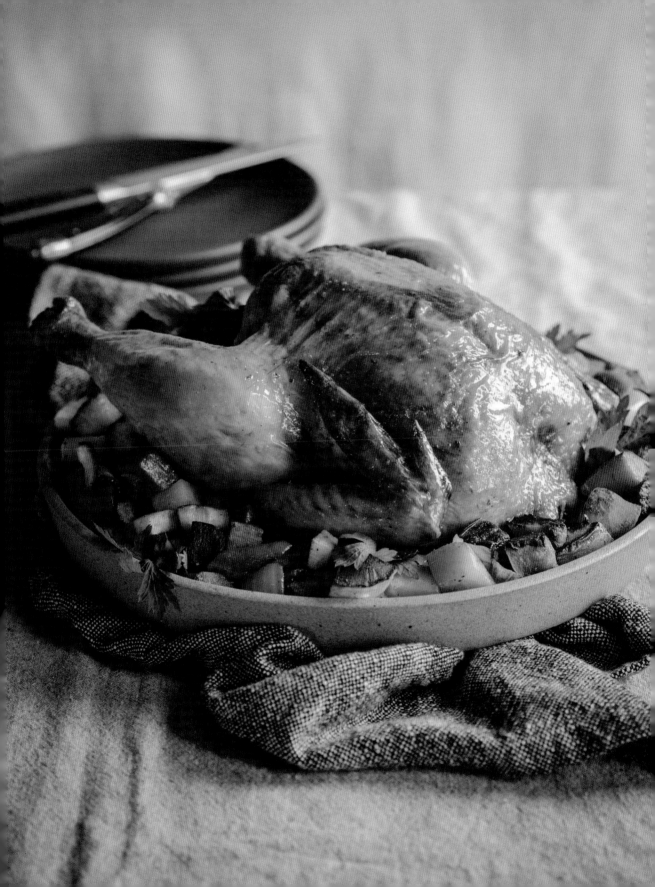

Whole Roasted Chicken
with Maple Root Vegetables

A whole roasted chicken is a weekly staple in our home. It's one of the most nourishing and easiest meals in this book. Remember, quality ingredients make simple food taste incredible, so don't skimp on your choice of chicken if possible. I prefer organic, pasture-raised, whole chicken for this recipe. SERVES 6-8

DF | GF

1 whole chicken (about 4 pounds)

Coarse sea salt and ground black pepper

2 medium red potatoes, chopped (about 2 cups)

2 large carrots, halved lengthwise and chopped (about 1 cup)

1 medium yellow onion, chopped (about 1 cup)

1 parsnip, chopped (about 1½ cups)

1 tablespoon olive oil

2 tablespoons maple syrup

¾ teaspoon sea salt

¼ teaspoon ground black pepper

Fresh parsley leaves, stems removed

Remove the chicken from the refrigerator and bring to room temperature before cooking, about 30 to 45 minutes. This will produce a juicier and more evenly cooked chicken. Position one oven rack in the middle of the oven and one below it; preheat oven to 400°F. Using paper towels, thoroughly dry your chicken on both sides and inside the carcass. The drier the skin before cooking, the crispier the skin after cooking. I do not truss my chicken, but feel free to do this if you prefer. Trussing can help the chicken cook and brown more evenly, but I find that it's unnecessary for smaller birds.

Liberally season both sides and the cavity of the chicken with coarse sea salt and pepper. Place the chicken in a rectangular 9" × 13" baking dish or on a baking sheet and roast for 50 to 60 minutes, or until the skin has turned a golden brown and the juices run clear or nearly clear (versus red or pink). You can use a meat thermometer if you prefer, removing the chicken when the internal temperature reaches 160°F to 165°F. The skin should be crispy enough at this point to make a distinctly crisp sound when tapped.

While the chicken is cooking, prepare your vegetables (removing the peels if they are nonorganic). Chop the vegetables all the same size to ensure they cook within the same time frame. Combine the chopped vegetables on a large baking sheet and add the olive oil, maple syrup, salt, and pepper. Toss to coat and set aside. After the chicken has cooked for 30 minutes, place the vegetables in the oven on the rack below the chicken. Cook them for 25 to 30 minutes or until fork tender and lightly browned. The chicken and vegetables should be done around the same time.

→

Reserve the chicken carcass, once the meat is removed, for making Bone Broth (page 100).

Remove the chicken and vegetables from the oven and let rest, loosely covered with a foil tent, for 10 to 15 minutes before carving. Do not seal your chicken with foil or the skin will soften and won't stay crispy. Once rested, carve your chicken. Pour the juices from the chicken pan over the roasted vegetables and stir. Place the chicken in the center of a large serving dish and arrange the vegetables around it, then garnish with parsley leaves. Serve warm.

Yellow Pumpkin Curry
with Toasted Cashews

This hearty vegan curry celebrates the humble and nourishing pumpkin while highlighting the immune-boosting and anti-inflammatory properties of pumpkin, fresh ginger, garlic, and turmeric. Fun fact: did you know that the terms *pumpkin* and *winter squash* can be used interchangeably for those beloved, starchy, vine-grown vegetables? SERVES 6

DF | GF | V | Ve

1 tablespoon coconut oil

1 medium white or yellow onion, chopped

3 large carrots, chopped

½ small sugar pumpkin or kabocha squash, peeled with seeds removed, cut into bitesize pieces

1 teaspoon sea salt

½ teaspoon ground black pepper

2 tablespoons fresh grated ginger

1 tablespoon minced garlic

2 teaspoons fresh grated turmeric

3 tablespoons yellow curry paste or Golden Turmeric Paste (page 103)

1 green bell pepper, sliced lengthwise

One 10- or 12-ounce bag frozen green peas

Two 13.5-ounce cans unsweetened full-fat coconut milk

½ cup whole raw cashews, toasted and roughly chopped

Fresh cilantro

1 lime, cut into wedges

Heat oil in a large sauté pan or skillet over medium heat. Add the onion, carrots, pumpkin, salt, and pepper; sauté until the onions are translucent, about 7 to 10 minutes. Add the ginger, garlic, turmeric, and yellow curry paste or Golden Turmeric Paste, and cook for an additional 30 seconds. Finally, add the bell pepper, peas, and coconut milk, stirring all ingredients together with a wooden spoon.

Increase the heat slightly and bring the curry to a gentle boil, stirring occasionally. Reduce the heat to a simmer and cook uncovered for an additional 20 minutes or until the pumpkin is fork tender (your cooking time will vary depending on the size of your pumpkin pieces). Once the pumpkin is cooked through, season to taste with additional salt as needed. Serve warm over cooked whole grains or with whole wheat flatbread, and garnish with cashews, fresh cilantro, and a squeeze of lime.

Loaded Sweet Potatoes
with Sautéed Kale and Onions

Loaded with your favorite ingredients, one of these sweet potatoes can easily become your next meal. Remember to eat the skin too for additional antioxidants, fiber, iron, protein, and various vitamins. Try other tasty topping combinations, such as finely chopped white onions, black beans, cheddar cheese, salsa, guacamole, and cilantro, or curried chickpeas, sautéed red onions, spinach, tahini, and lime. MAKES 4 SWEET POTATOES

DF | GF | V | Ve

SWEET POTATOES

4 large organic sweet potatoes (skin on), washed well

1 tablespoon olive oil or butter

Sea salt and ground black pepper

TOPPINGS

1+ tablespoon olive oil or butter

1 medium yellow onion, halved and sliced thin (about 1 cup)

¼ teaspoon sea salt

1 bunch kale, stems discarded and leaves chopped into thin ribbons (about 3–4 cups)

1 cup cooked or canned black beans, drained and rinsed

3 tablespoons chopped chives

¼ cup plain whole milk yogurt or sour cream, or plant-based alternative

Place one oven rack in the middle of your oven and one just below it; preheat oven to 400°F. Place a baking sheet lined with foil on the lower rack to catch any drippings that may be produced while cooking the sweet potatoes directly on the rack above.

Using fork tines, poke numerous holes in each sweet potato. These will act as vents to release steam when cooking. Oil or butter the outside of each potato and season liberally with salt and pepper. Place the potatoes directly on the oven rack above the baking sheet and bake for 60 to 90 minutes, depending on the size of your potatoes. After 60 minutes, you can cut a small slit with a knife into one of the larger potatoes and assess for doneness. The interior should be soft with no hard lumps and the skin slightly crispy.

Meanwhile, start your toppings. Add 1 tablespoon olive oil or butter to a large sauté pan over medium to high heat. Add the onion and salt, and sauté for 7 to 9 minutes or until the onion is translucent and tender. Add the kale and sauté for an additional 2 to 3 minutes or until the kale has softened and reduced in size. Add a splash of water to your sauté pan, if necessary, to tenderize the kale even more and to deglaze your pan. Remove from the heat and set aside. Place all other topping ingredients in assembly-line fashion awaiting the hot potatoes.

Once the potatoes are done cooking, remove from the oven and let cool slightly on a cooling rack for about 10 minutes, or until cool enough to handle. Using a sharp knife, cut a slit down the center of each potato and squeeze the ends together, opening the potatoes wide for toppings. Using a fork, mash the interior of each potato and help the flesh release from the edges before adding the toppings. Serve warm.

Spiced Whole Wheat Ginger and Molasses Cookies

These make for the best seasonal cookies during the holidays. The blackstrap molasses provides notable amounts of calcium, magnesium, potassium, selenium, manganese, and copper. Always use blackstrap molasses versus light or dark molasses to ensure the highest nutrient content possible, and choose unsulphured molasses to minimize the environmental impact of sugar cane and molasses production and to avoid the addition of sulfur dioxide, a potentially harmful additive used to extend the shelf life. MAKES 2 DOZEN COOKIES

V

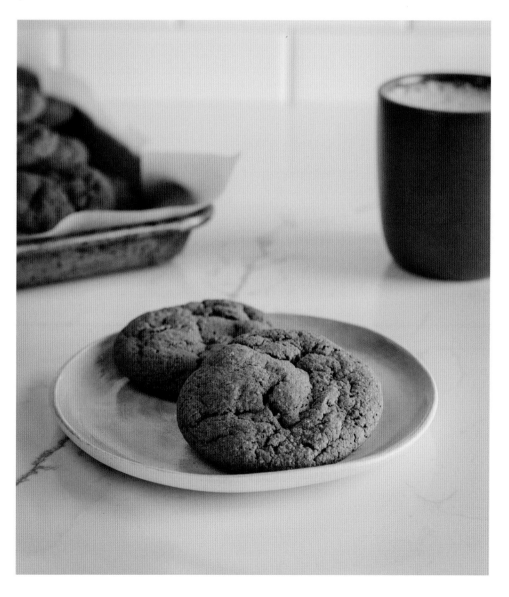

2½ cups whole wheat
  pastry flour

2 teaspoons baking soda

1 tablespoon ground ginger

1½ teaspoons ground cinnamon

1 teaspoon ground cardamom

½ teaspoon ground cloves

½ teaspoon sea salt

½ pound unsalted butter
  (2 sticks), softened

¾ cup maple sugar or unrefined
  coconut sugar

1 egg

½ cup blackstrap molasses

2 tablespoons finely grated
  fresh ginger

Position the oven racks in the middle of the oven, and pre-heat oven to 350°F. Line two baking sheets with parchment paper and set aside.

In a large bowl, whisk the flour, baking soda, ginger, cin-namon, cardamom, cloves, and sea salt together. Set aside. In an electric stand mixer fitted with a whisk attachment or separate large bowl with a handheld electric mixer, cream the butter and maple or coconut sugar together until light and fluffy. Add the egg and beat until combined. Add the molasses and combine thoroughly. Slowly add the flour mix-ture to the wet ingredients, mixing on low speed until just combined. Your dough should be light and soft to the touch. Add the fresh ginger and mix again on low speed for 10 to 15 seconds until the ginger is evenly dispersed.

With clean hands, roll dough to golf ball–size balls and place them on the baking sheets, spacing them at least 2 inches apart (they will spread). It's OK if the balls are not perfectly round, as they will flatten symmetrically as they bake.

Bake the cookies for a total of 10 to 12 minutes, switching the bottom baking sheet to the top and vice versa half-way through, which will allow the cookies to bake evenly. Alternatively, you can bake one cookie sheet at a time, while storing the remaining cookie dough in the refrigerator. The tops of the cookies will form those quintessential ginger molasses cookie cracks when they're done. Remove from the oven and let cool completely before enjoying with your favorite warm beverage.

You can freeze the cookie dough before baking in a tightly sealed freezer bag for 3 months. Thaw the cookie dough in the refrigerator for 24 to 48 hours before baking.

Dark Chocolate Banana Bread
with Toasted Almonds

The dark chocolate and toasted almonds make this bread more swoon-worthy than your typical banana bread. Did you know that dark chocolate is actually a powerful antioxidant? Consuming small amounts regularly has been associated with a lower risk of heart disease and strokes. SERVES 10

V

4 ripe or overripe bananas

¼ cup dark brown sugar

¼ cup honey

2 eggs

1 teaspoon vanilla extract

½ cup whole milk, room temperature or slightly warm

½ cup coconut oil, melted

1¾ cups whole wheat flour

1 teaspoon baking soda

½ teaspoon sea salt

¼ teaspoon ground cinnamon

One 3- to 4-ounce bar 60%–70% cacao dark chocolate, roughly chopped

¼ cup raw almonds, chopped

2 tablespoons sliced almonds

Preheat oven to 350°F. Oil a 9-inch loaf pan with coconut oil and set aside. Using clean hands or the back of a fork, mash the bananas in a medium-size bowl. Add the brown sugar, honey, eggs, vanilla, milk, and melted coconut oil; whisk until smooth. In a separate bowl, whisk together the dry ingredients except the chocolate and almonds. Using a rubber spatula, mix the dry and wet ingredients together until just combined. Fold in the chocolate and chopped almonds (not sliced almonds).

Pour the batter into the loaf pan and use your spatula to even out the top. Sprinkle the sliced almonds on top. Bake for 50 to 60 minutes, or until a knife inserted in the center comes out clean. The almonds on top should be toasted and golden brown. Remove from the oven and allow the loaf to cool for at least 5 minutes before removing the whole loaf from the pan and placing on a cooling rack. Let it cool completely to room temperature before slicing and serving.

You can freeze the whole loaf or individual slices (after baking) for 2 to 3 months. If freezing, wrap room-temperature banana bread in plastic wrap before wrapping it in foil or storing in a resealable freezer bag.

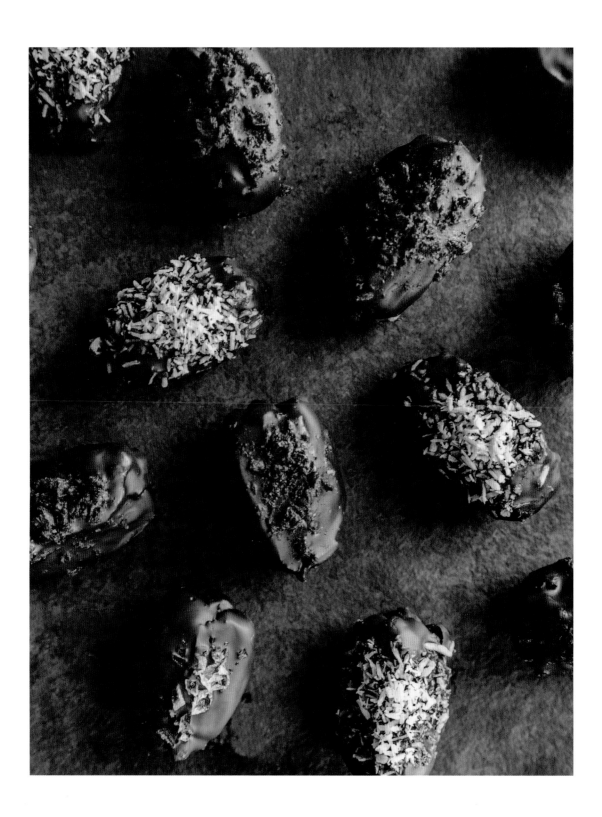

Cashew Butter Stuffed Dates
with Dark Chocolate and Sea Salt

This is one of the fastest and most satisfying desserts I know! Your family and friends will be begging you to make more. Dates make for a great snack or dessert on the go. Substitute whole raw or roasted nuts for the nut butter for a crunchy twist and/or play with various toppings like shredded coconut flakes, crushed dehydrated raspberries, fresh orange zest, or finely chopped nuts. **MAKES 12 STUFFED DATES**

DF | GF | V | Ve | RT

One 3- to 4-ounce bar 60%–70% cacao dark chocolate, roughly chopped

2 teaspoons coconut oil

12 large pitted dates

¼ cup cashew or alternative nut butter

Large-flake sea salt or Maldon sea salt or other toppings

In a double boiler over medium heat, melt the chocolate and coconut oil together, stirring regularly with a rubber spatula. While these ingredients are melting, line a baking sheet with parchment paper and set aside.

Cut each date open like a book with a small sharp knife, making one cut lengthwise on one side of the date. You don't want to cut all the way through the date, although it's an easy fix if you do. Using a spoon, scoop about 1 teaspoon of nut butter (or filling of choice) into the center of each sliced date and gently squeeze the date closed. If you accidently cut through the entire date, place nut butter in the center, sandwiching the date pieces back together. It's OK if there's nut butter squeezing out the sides or stuck to the outside of the date. This recipe is very forgiving—everything eventually gets covered in chocolate and disappears (what a dream!). Add nut butter to all the dates and place on the prepared baking sheet.

The chocolate mixture should be completely melted by now. Turn off the double boiler. Place dates, one at a time, in the melted chocolate mixture and roll them around with a fork, covering all sides with melted chocolate. Gently lift each date out with the fork and place on the baking sheet to cool. Spoon additional chocolate onto any exposed areas if necessary. Finish covering all the dates with chocolate, then add a pinch of large-flake or Maldon sea salt (or your topping of choice) to each date. Finally, place the baking sheet in the refrigerator for 45 minutes or until the chocolate cools completely and solidifies. Serve cold or bring individual servings to room temperature for about 10 minutes before serving. If left out at room temperature for too long, they will begin to sweat.

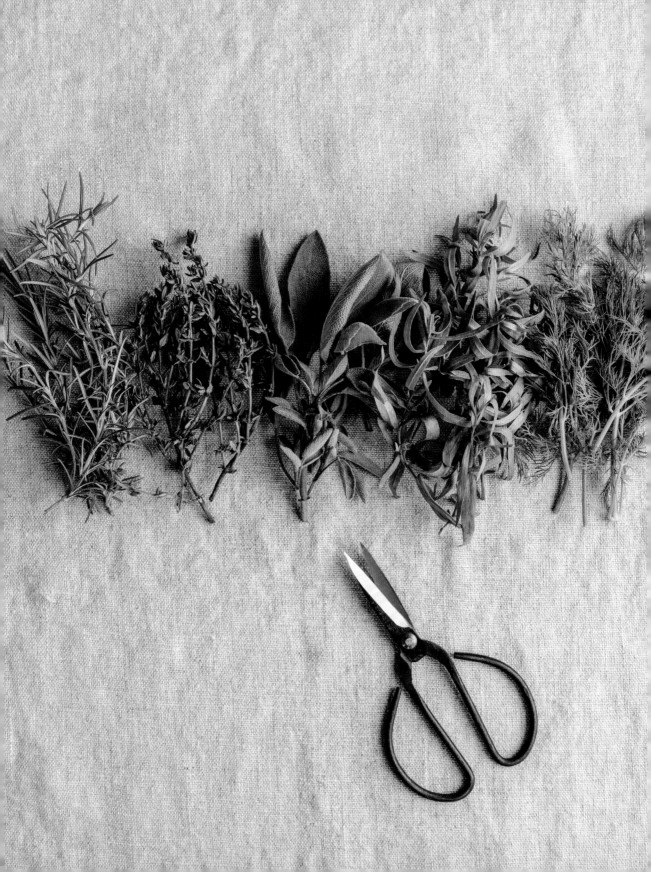

SEASONAL MEAL PLANS

Learning to eat a seasonal whole foods diet can feel overwhelming at first, especially if it's a big leap from your current diet. To help you get started, and to make the transition easier, I've created a sample three-day meal plan or menu for each of the four seasons. Try one or all of them—just remember to start with the current season for the freshest flavors, maximum nutrients, and most readily available ingredients.

Most recipes in each meal plan make at least two to four servings, if not more, so be sure to read through the recipe in advance and adjust your ingredients as needed for your household. I've considered which meals make great (and effortless) leftovers and repeat some or all of the recipes on multiple days within the same meal plan for convenience and to save you time and money when possible. This doesn't mean you cook the same recipe twice; rather, you make the recipe once when it first appears, and the portions will cover you for the subsequent meal as well, sometimes with a slight tweak or twist (for example, Chicken Meatballs with Basil Walnut Pesto served on salad greens one day and on whole wheat spaghetti noodles another). Finally, I offer three snack options for every meal plan, using the surplus from the recipes, as well as one delicious dessert.

I have also included shopping lists for each menu, so you can give this a try without any additional work or stress. Make sure you compare the shopping list to your current pantry and fridge/freezer before shopping to minimize waste and duplication, and review each recipe for further guidance before starting your food prep or cooking.

Bon appetit!

Three-Day Spring Meal Plan

	DAY 1	DAY 2	DAY 3
Breakfast	Strawberry Vanilla Almond Butter Smoothie with Bee Pollen (page 121)	Baby Spinach and Spring Onion Frittata with Goat Cheese (page 122) + oven-roasted baby potatoes (olive oil, potatoes, salt/pepper)	Strawberry Vanilla Almond Butter Smoothie with Bee Pollen (page 121)
Lunch	Vegetable Miso Soup with Kombu Dashi and Tofu (page 126) Spicy Sriracha Mung Bean Bowl with Pickled Daikon and Carrots (page 127)	Chicken Meatballs with Basil Walnut Pesto (page 132) + green salad with fresh cherries	Baby Spinach and Spring Onion Frittata with Goat Cheese (page 122) Butter-Roasted Radishes with Radish Greens (page 123)
Dinner	Chicken Meatballs with Basil Walnut Pesto (page 132) + whole wheat spaghetti (olive oil, spaghetti, s/p)	Vegetable Miso Soup with Kombu Dashi and Tofu (page 126) + long-grain brown rice (make additional rice for dinner tomorrow) + avocado slices	Vegetable Fried Brown Rice with Ginger Sauce (page 133)

SNACKS

Red bell pepper and carrot sticks with pesto
Plain Whole Milk Yogurt (page 110) or store-
    bought yogurt of choice with strawberries
    and sweetener (optional)
Pecans and walnuts

DESSERT

Strawberry Rhubarb Crisp (page 139)

Spring Shopping List

PANTRY STAPLES

Check your pantry for these ingredients before shopping.

- [ ] Vanilla extract
- [ ] Cold-pressed extra virgin olive oil
- [ ] Toasted sesame oil
- [ ] Tamari or soy sauce
- [ ] Honey
- [ ] Rice wine vinegar
- [ ] Sriracha
- [ ] Red wine vinegar
- [ ] Avocado oil
- [ ] White wine vinegar
- [ ] Fine sea salt
- [ ] Black pepper
- [ ] 1 (16 oz.) glass jar with lid

PRODUCE

- [ ] 2 bananas
- [ ] 1 garlic bulb
- [ ] 1 bunch parsley (curly or flat leaf)
- [ ] 2⅓ cups basil
- [ ] 6 large carrots
- [ ] 1 bunch celery
- [ ] 1 head green cabbage
- [ ] 4 inches fresh ginger
- [ ] 2–3 ounces fresh enoki mushrooms
- [ ] 1 cup shiitake mushrooms
- [ ] 2 bunches scallions
- [ ] 1 medium daikon radish
- [ ] 1 small Napa cabbage
- [ ] ½ small red cabbage
- [ ] 1 cucumber
- [ ] 2 avocados
- [ ] 1 bunch cilantro
- [ ] 4 cups baby spinach
- [ ] 1 pound baby potatoes
- [ ] Salad greens
- [ ] 2 bunches radishes (with greens)
- [ ] 1 lemon
- [ ] 1 white onion
- [ ] 1 red bell pepper
- [ ] 1 head broccoli
- [ ] 1½ pounds fresh strawberries
- [ ] ½ pound rhubarb
- [ ] ½ pound cherries

REFRIGERATOR/FREEZER

- [ ] 2 cups frozen strawberries
- [ ] 3 cups plant-based milk
- [ ] Bee pollen (optional)
- [ ] 1 cup whole-milk ricotta
- [ ] 2-ounce wedge parmesan cheese
- [ ] 1 (8 oz.) container white miso paste
- [ ] 8 ounces firm tofu
- [ ] 8 ounces sour cream or plant-based alternative
- [ ] 32 ounces plain whole-milk yogurt or plant-based alternative
- [ ] 14 eggs (or 6–8 oz. extra-firm tofu)
- [ ] ½ cup whole milk
- [ ] 2 ounces plain soft goat cheese
- [ ] 2 sticks butter
- [ ] 1 (10–12 oz.) bag frozen green peas

POULTRY/MEAT/SEAFOOD

- [ ] 2 pounds ground dark meat chicken (or mixture of dark and white meat)

CANNED/BOTTLED/DRY GOODS

- [ ] 6 tablespoons almond butter
- [ ] 4–6 pitted dates
- [ ] ⅓ cup walnuts
- [ ] 1 (14.5 oz.) box whole wheat spaghetti
- [ ] 2 cups short-grain brown rice
- [ ] 2½ cups long-grain brown rice
- [ ] 1 cup sprouted dried mung beans
- [ ] 1 package dried kombu seaweed
- [ ] 1 package dried wakame seaweed
- [ ] 1 small jar chili oil
- [ ] 1 small bottle mirin
- [ ] 1 cup rolled oats
- [ ] ⅔ cup finely ground almond flour
- [ ] ½ cup Sucanat or coconut sugar
- [ ] ⅔ cup pecans
- [ ] ⅔ cup walnuts

DRIED HERBS/SPICES

- [ ] Garlic powder
- [ ] Black sesame seeds
- [ ] Ground cinnamon
- [ ] Nutmeg
- [ ] Arrowroot powder

Three-Day Summer Meal Plan

	DAY 1	DAY 2	DAY 3
Breakfast	Sweet Cornmeal Pancakes with Vanilla Roasted Peaches (page 145) + Plain Whole Milk Yogurt (page 110) or store-bought yogurt of choice	Egg Muffins with Tomato Salsa and Lime-Marinated Avocado (page 144) + tortillas of choice	Egg Muffins with Tomato Salsa and Lime-Marinated Avocado (page 144) + Whole Wheat and Flax Tortillas (page 157)
Lunch	Rainbow Rolls with Ginger Almond Sauce (page 141)	Salmon en Papillote with Seasonal Vegetable Ribbons (page 159) + sautéed zucchini noodles (olive oil, zucchini noodles, salt/pepper)	Rainbow Rolls with Ginger Almond Sauce (page 141) + grilled chicken breasts or tofu (olive oil, chicken/tofu, salt/pepper)
Dinner	Quinoa Tabbouleh with Roasted Cherry Tomatoes (page 151) + grilled chicken breasts or tofu (olive oil, chicken/tofu, salt/pepper)	The Simplest Tempeh Tacos (page 155) + Whole Wheat and Flax Tortillas (page 157), or whole grain tortillas	Salmon en Papillote with Seasonal Vegetable Ribbons (page 159) + sautéed green beans (butter, green beans, lemon juice, salt/pepper)

SNACKS
Cultured Key Lime Cashew Yogurt (page 143)
Plain Whole Milk Yogurt (page 110) or store-
　　bought yogurt of choice and peach slices
Hard-boiled egg(s) and cucumber sticks

DESSERT
Blueberry Acai and Coconut Ice Pops (page 163)

Summary Shopping List

PANTRY STAPLES

Check your pantry for these ingredients before shopping.

- [ ] Baking powder
- [ ] Fine sea salt
- [ ] Black pepper
- [ ] Maple syrup
- [ ] Vanilla extract
- [ ] Toasted sesame oil
- [ ] Tamari or soy sauce
- [ ] Honey
- [ ] Cold-pressed extra virgin olive oil
- [ ] Avocado oil
- [ ] 4 (8 oz.) glass jars with lids
- [ ] Cheesecloth
- [ ] 6–8 ice pop molds

PRODUCE

- [ ] 3 peaches
- [ ] 1 bunch rainbow chard
- [ ] 1 medium red cabbage
- [ ] 1 yellow bell pepper
- [ ] 2 English cucumbers
- [ ] 3 large carrots
- [ ] 3 bunches cilantro
- [ ] 2 limes
- [ ] 1 inch fresh ginger
- [ ] 1 garlic bulb
- [ ] 1 pint cherry tomatoes
- [ ] 3 medium vine-ripened or Roma tomatoes
- [ ] 1 bunch scallions
- [ ] 1 bunch curly parsley
- [ ] 1 bunch flat leaf parsley
- [ ] 1 handful mint
- [ ] 3 lemons
- [ ] 1 yellow onion
- [ ] 1 red bell pepper
- [ ] 1 green bell pepper
- [ ] 2 avocadoes
- [ ] 1 small zucchini
- [ ] 20 ounces zucchini noodles (or 4 zucchinis)
- [ ] 1 bunch spinach
- [ ] 1 white onion
- [ ] 1 pound green beans
- [ ] 16–18 key limes

REFRIGERATOR/FREEZER

- [ ] 18 eggs
- [ ] ½ cup whole milk or plant-based alternative
- [ ] 1 stick butter
- [ ] 24 ounces yogurt of choice (or Plain Whole Milk Yogurt)
- [ ] ¼ cup crumbled queso fresco
- [ ] 24 ounces fresh tomato salsa
- [ ] 12 ounces organic soy tempeh
- [ ] ¼ cup shredded cheddar cheese
- [ ] 1½ cups cashew milk
- [ ] 2 (10–15 billion CFU) probiotic capsules
- [ ] ½ cup fresh or frozen blueberries
- [ ] 1 (3–4 oz.) package frozen unsweetened acai purée

POULTRY/MEAT/SEAFOOD

- [ ] 2–4 chicken breasts or 8 ounces firm tofu
- [ ] 4 (4 oz.) salmon fillets

CANNED/BOTTLED/DRY GOODS

- [ ] 1½ cups whole-grain oat flour
- [ ] 1 cup medium grind whole-grain yellow cornmeal
- [ ] 1 (8 oz.) package dried thin rice noodles or vermicelli noodles
- [ ] ½ cup almond butter
- [ ] ⅔ cup white quinoa
- [ ] 24 whole-grain tortillas (or Whole Wheat and Flax Tortillas)
- [ ] 2 cups raw unsalted cashews
- [ ] 1 (13.5 oz.) can coconut cream or full-fat coconut milk

DRIED HERBS/SPICES

- [ ] Red chili flakes
- [ ] Cumin
- [ ] Coriander
- [ ] Cayenne

Three-Day Autumn Meal Plan

	DAY 1	DAY 2	DAY 3
Breakfast	Roasted Banana and Almond Butter Breakfast Cookies (page 167)	Cinnamon Apple Overnight Oats with Toasted Walnuts (page 168)	Roasted Banana and Almond Butter Breakfast Cookies (page 167)
Lunch	Wheat Berry Salad with Butternut Squash and Maple Vinaigrette (page 173) (make additional wheat berries for dinner tomorrow) Mirin and Miso Glazed Cod (page 178)	Broccoli Salad with Pickled Cranberries and Herb Yogurt Dressing (page 169) Coconut Curry Red Lentil Stew with Cilantro Lime Chutney (page 175)	Beef and Beet Borscht with Fresh Beet Greens (page 181) + sourdough rye bread with butter
Dinner	Broccoli Salad with Pickled Cranberries and Herb Yogurt Dressing (page 169) Beef and Beet Borscht with Fresh Beet Greens (page 181) + sourdough rye bread with butter	Mirin and Miso-Glazed Cod (page 178) + wheat berries + roasted baby bok choy (baby bok choy, toasted sesame oil, tamari or soy sauce)	Coconut Curry Red Lentil Stew with Cilantro Lime Chutney (page 175) + whole wheat pita

SNACKS

Sourdough rye bread or whole wheat pita
    with hummus
Apple slices and almond butter
Popcorn, coconut oil, and nutritional yeast

DESSERT

Chocolate Tofu Mousse with Coconut Whip
(page 182)

Autumn Shopping List

PANTRY STAPLES

Check your pantry for these ingredients
before shopping.

- ☐ Maple syrup
- ☐ Baking powder
- ☐ Baking soda
- ☐ Fine sea salt
- ☐ Black pepper
- ☐ Coconut oil
- ☐ Vanilla extract
- ☐ Cold-pressed extra virgin olive oil
- ☐ Apple cider vinegar
- ☐ Toasted sesame oil
- ☐ Honey
- ☐ Tamari or soy sauce
- ☐ 8 (8 oz.) or 4 (16 oz.) glass jars with lids

PRODUCE

- ☐ 2 bananas
- ☐ 1 butternut squash
- ☐ 2 red onions
- ☐ 1 bunch flat-leaf parsley
- ☐ 2 broccoli heads
- ☐ 1 handful fresh tarragon
- ☐ 6 red beets (with greens)
- ☐ 2 yellow onions
- ☐ 2 large carrots
- ☐ 4 small apples
- ☐ 1 bunch spinach
- ☐ 1 bunch cilantro
- ☐ 1 bunch scallions
- ☐ 1 lime
- ☐ 4 baby bok choy

REFRIGERATOR/FREEZER

- ☐ 1 (8 oz.) container white miso
- ☐ 24 ounces plain yogurt (or Plain Whole Milk Yogurt)
- ☐ ⅓ cup blue cheese
- ☐ 1 stick butter
- ☐ 3 cups whole milk or plant-based alternative
- ☐ 1 (8–10 oz.) container hummus
- ☐ 1 (12–14 oz.) container silken tofu

POULTRY/MEAT/SEAFOOD

- ☐ 6 (6 oz.) skinless cod fillets
- ☐ 2 pounds boneless beef short ribs or chuck roast

CANNED/BOTTLED/DRY GOODS

- ☐ 1 cup quinoa flakes
- ☐ 2 cups superfine almond flour
- ☐ 2 cups almond butter
- ☐ ¼ cup raw almonds
- ☐ ¾ cup raw walnuts
- ☐ 2½ cups wheat berries
- ☐ 1 cup dried cranberries
- ☐ 1 small bottle mirin
- ☐ ½ cup sliced almonds
- ☐ 2½ quarts low-sodium beef stock
- ☐ 1 small jar whole-grain mustard
- ☐ 1 small loaf sourdough rye bread
- ☐ 3 cups rolled oats
- ☐ 2 tablespoons chia seeds
- ☐ 1 (28 oz.) can diced tomatoes
- ☐ 3 (13.5 oz.) cans full-fat coconut milk or coconut cream
- ☐ 4 cups vegetable broth
- ☐ 1½ cups red lentils
- ☐ 1 package whole wheat pita
- ☐ ½ cup popcorn kernels
- ☐ Unsweetened cacao powder
- ☐ ¼ cup large coconut flakes (optional)
- ☐ Raw cacao nibs (optional)

DRIED HERBS/SPICES

- ☐ Ground cinnamon
- ☐ Ground ginger
- ☐ Ground nutmeg
- ☐ Ground turmeric
- ☐ Cumin
- ☐ Ground cardamom
- ☐ Cayenne
- ☐ 1 whole cinnamon stick
- ☐ Nutritional yeast

Three-Day Winter Meal Plan

	DAY 1	DAY 2	DAY 3
Breakfast	Buckwheat Breakfast Porridge with Cranberry Chia Compote (page 191)	Homemade Whole Wheat Toaster Waffles (page 188) + nut butter and fruit jam	Buckwheat Breakfast Porridge with Cranberry Chia Compote (page 191)
Lunch	Spicy Three Bean Chili (page 197) + guacamole + tricolor quinoa	Curly Kale and Wild Rice Salad with Sweet Fennel and Garlic Vinaigrette (page 195) Spicy Three Bean Chili (page 197)	Roasted Brussel Sprouts with Honey Miso Glaze and Cilantro (page 199) + fried or soft-boiled egg(s) + kasha or buckwheat
Dinner	Curly Kale and Wild Rice Salad with Sweet Fennel and Garlic Vinaigrette (page 195) Whole Roasted Chicken with Maple Root Vegetables (page 201)	Whole Roasted Chicken with Maple Root Vegetables (page 201) + sautéed chard (olive oil, chard, salt/pepper)	Yellow Pumpkin Curry with Toasted Cashews (page 203) + long-grain brown rice + sautéed kale (ghee, kale, salt/pepper)

SNACKS

Bone Broth (page 100) or store-bought
  alternative

Plain Whole Milk Yogurt (page 110) or
  store-bought yogurt and **Cranberry Chia
  Compote** (page 191)

Cashews and banana

DESSERT

**Spiced Whole Wheat Ginger and
  Molasses Cookies** (page 205)

Winter Shopping List

PANTRY STAPLES

Check your pantry for these ingredients before shopping.

- [ ] Cold-pressed extra virgin olive oil
- [ ] Fine sea salt
- [ ] Black pepper
- [ ] Maple syrup
- [ ] Coarse sea salt
- [ ] Maple syrup
- [ ] Vanilla extract
- [ ] Baking soda
- [ ] Toasted sesame oil
- [ ] Honey
- [ ] Rice wine vinegar
- [ ] Coconut oil

PRODUCE

- [ ] 2 yellow onions
- [ ] 2 green bell peppers
- [ ] 2 poblano peppers
- [ ] 2 jalapeño peppers
- [ ] 2 garlic bulbs
- [ ] 2 limes
- [ ] 1 fennel bulb
- [ ] 1 bunch curly kale
- [ ] 1 bunch rainbow chard
- [ ] 1 bunch flat-leaf parsley
- [ ] 2 lemons
- [ ] 2 medium red potatoes
- [ ] 5 large carrots
- [ ] 1 parsnip
- [ ] 1½ pounds brussel sprouts
- [ ] 1 bunch cilantro
- [ ] 1 white onion
- [ ] 1 small sugar pumpkin or kabocha squash
- [ ] 2 tablespoons fresh turmeric
- [ ] 1 bunch kale
- [ ] 2 bananas
- [ ] 2 inches ginger
- [ ] 1 orange

REFRIGERATOR/FREEZER

- [ ] 10–12 ounces fresh or frozen cranberries
- [ ] 1 medium orange
- [ ] 4 inches fresh ginger
- [ ] 20 ounces whole milk or plant-based alternative
- [ ] 16 ounces plain whole-milk yogurt or plant-based alternative
- [ ] 1 (8 oz.) container guacamole or 8 ounces homemade guacamole
- [ ] 3 sticks butter
- [ ] 6 eggs
- [ ] 1 (8 oz.) container white miso
- [ ] 1 (10–12 oz.) bag frozen green peas
- [ ] Bone broth (store-bought or homemade)

POULTRY/MEAT/SEAFOOD

- [ ] 1 (4 lb.) whole chicken

CANNED/BOTTLED/DRY GOODS

- [ ] 1½ cups raw buckwheat groats
- [ ] 1½ cups tricolor quinoa
- [ ] 2 tablespoons chia seeds
- [ ] 2 tablespoons raw pumpkin seeds
- [ ] ½ cup dried cranberries
- [ ] ¾ cup dried pinto beans
- [ ] ¾ cup dried kidney beans
- [ ] ¾ cup dried black beans
- [ ] 2 (14–15 oz.) cans diced tomatoes
- [ ] 1 (14–15 oz.) can tomato sauce
- [ ] 1 quart vegetable stock
- [ ] 1 cup wild rice
- [ ] 1 package or small jar active dry yeast
- [ ] 4½ cups whole wheat pastry flour
- [ ] Nut butter of choice (optional)
- [ ] Fruit jam of choice (optional)
- [ ] 1 small bottle fish sauce
- [ ] 1 small jar yellow curry paste (or Golden Turmeric Paste)
- [ ] 2 (13.5 oz.) cans full-fat coconut milk
- [ ] 1½ cups raw whole cashews
- [ ] 1 cup long-grain brown rice
- [ ] 1 small jar ghee
- [ ] ¾ cup maple sugar or unrefined coconut sugar
- [ ] ½ cup blackstrap molasses

DRIED HERBS/SPICES

- [ ] Chili powder
- [ ] Oregano
- [ ] Cumin
- [ ] Cayenne
- [ ] 8 whole cardamom pods
- [ ] 1 whole cinnamon stick
- [ ] Ground ginger
- [ ] Ground cinnamon
- [ ] Ground cloves
- [ ] Ground cardamom

ACKNOWLEDGMENTS

With love and gratitude, I want to acknowledge everyone who helped create this book.

My son, August Knowles: Thank you for infusing me with creative energy—you are my greatest creation! I look forward to the day when you and I can play in the kitchen together. My beloved husband, partner, and the best dishwasher I know, Tom Knowles: Thank you for supporting me on this unconventional and circuitous path. Your endless love gives me the strength and courage to keep reaching for the stars. My supportive parents, Chuck and Trish Kellogg: For always making my dreams and goals, even the wildest ones, feel attainable. Thank you. My dearest sister, Hilly Shue: You constantly inspire me in the most beautiful ways and challenge me to think outside the box. Thank you for being a gentle and compassionate guide and teacher. Patty Kellogg, proofreader and editor extraordinaire: Thank you for dedicating so much time to my manuscript.

Dr. JJ Pursell, my colleague, mentor, and friend: Thank you for believing in me and providing me with this incredible opportunity. Cari Sanchez-Potter, the ultimate boss babe and recipe-testing goddess: You are a good friend. Thank you for the incredible feedback! My dear friend, Cecily Read: Thank you for your generosity and time in recipe testing. The Shah family: Thank you for offering up your gorgeous home and kitchen for this project! My good friend and colleague, Dr. Erin Conlon: Thank you for your critical and scientific eye. Serena Stearns-Garland, assistant and friend: Thank you for volunteering your time. Seasonal recipe testers and proofreaders: Thank you for your support and constructive feedback!

Sara Bercholz, Juree Sondker, Kara Plikaitis, Audra Figgins, Claire Kelley, Emma Hawkins, Karen Steib, Victoria Jones, Laura Shaw, and the entire Shambhala team: Thank you for giving this nutritionist a chance, for helping me find my voice and vision, and for turning my dream into a reality. I am incredibly grateful for your time and expertise. I will remember this experience (writing my first book!) for the rest of my life. Kimberley Hasselbrink, photographer: Thank you for the stunning images! You truly are the textile queen.

My Peruvian friends and family: Thank you for teaching me so much. Because of you, I found my calling. My teachers and community at Bastyr University: Thank you for sharing your knowledge of food and nutrition with me. My foundation and understanding of food as medicine started with you, and I'm so thankful it did. My dedicated and courageous patients: Without you, I would be certain of so much less. Endless thanks to you all.

Finally, to all of you reading and cooking from this book: Thank you for supporting my dream! I am forever grateful to you.

xx, Carly

APPENDIX A

Seasonal Produce Chart

FRUIT OR VEGETABLE	Freezer-Friendly	Available Canned	JANUARY	FEBRUARY	MARCH	APRIL	MAY	JUNE	JULY	AUGUST	SEPTEMBER	OCTOBER	NOVEMBER	DECEMBER
Apples		X									●	●	●	
Beets	X	X								●	●	●	●	
Bell peppers	X	X						●	●	●				
Blueberries	X							●	●					
Broccoli	X	X				●					●	●		
Cabbage		X			●	●								
Carrots	X	X								●	●	●		
Cauliflower	X										●	●		
Cherries	X	X						●	●					
Collard greens	X	X	●	●										●
Corn	X	X							●	●				
Cucumbers								●	●	●				
Eggplants									●	●	●			
Garlic								●	●	●	●	●	●	
Grapefruit		X	●	●										●
Grapes								●	●	●	●			
Lettuce/greens					●	●	●							
Kiwi			●	●										●

Source: www.fruitsandveggiesmorematters.org

FRUIT OR VEGETABLE	Freezer-Friendly	Available Canned	JANUARY	FEBRUARY	MARCH	APRIL	MAY	JUNE	JULY	AUGUST	SEPTEMBER	OCTOBER	NOVEMBER	DECEMBER
Melons								●	●	●				
Mushrooms	X	X	●	●	●	●					●	●	●	●
Onions	X		●	●	●	●	●							
Oranges		X	●	●										●
Parsnips											●	●	●	
Peaches	X	X						●	●	●				
Pears		X	●								●	●		
Plums								●	●	●	●			
Potatoes		X	●											●
Raspberries	X							●	●					
Spinach	X	X			●	●								
Strawberries	X						●	●						
Summer squash								●	●	●				
Sweet potatoes		X	●								●	●	●	
Tomatoes		X							●	●	●			
Turnips			●	●							●	●	●	●
Winter squash	X		●								●	●	●	●

APPENDIX B

Dietary Reference Intakes (DRI): Recommended Daily Allowances (RDA) and Adequate Intakes (AI)

Macronutrients

LIFE STAGE GROUP	TOTAL WATER (L)	CARBOHYDRATE (g)	TOTAL FIBER (g)
Infants			
0–6 mo	0.7	60	—
7–12 mo	0.8	95	—
Children			
1–3 y	1.3	130	19
4–8 y	1.7	130	25
Males			
9–13 y	2.4	130	31
14–18 y	3.3	130	38
19–30 y	3.7	130	38
31–50 y	3.7	130	38
51–70 y	3.7	130	30
>70 y	3.7	130	30
Females			
9–13 y	2.1	130	26
14–18 y	2.3	130	26
19–30 y	2.7	130	25
31–50 y	2.7	130	25
51–70 y	2.7	130	21
>70 y	2.7	130	21
Pregnancy			
14–18 y	3.0	175	28
19–30 y	3.0	175	28
31–50 y	3.0	175	28
Lactation			
14–18 y	3.8	210	29
19–30 y	3.8	210	29
31–50 y	3.8	210	29

Source: Food and Nutrition Board, Institute of Medicine, National Academies

FAT (g)	LINOLEIC ACID (g)	ALPHA-LINOLENIC ACID (g)	PROTEIN (g)
31	4.4	0.5	9.1
30	4.6	0.5	11.0
—	7	0.7	13
—	10	0.9	19
—	12	1.2	34
—	16	1.6	52
—	17	1.6	56
—	17	1.6	56
—	14	1.6	56
—	14	1.6	56
—	10	1.0	34
—	11	1.1	46
—	12	1.1	46
—	12	1.1	46
—	11	1.1	46
—	11	1.1	46
—	13	1.4	71
—	13	1.4	71
—	13	1.4	71
—	13	1.3	71
—	13	1.3	71
—	13	1.3	71

Vitamin Micronutrients

LIFE STAGE GROUP	VITAMIN A (μ/d)	VITAMIN C (mg/d)	VITAMIN D (μ/d)	VITAMIN E (mg/d)	VITAMIN K (μ/d)	THIAMIN (mg/d)
Infants						
0–6 mo	400	40	10	4	2.0	0.2
7–12 mo	500	50	10	5	2.5	0.3
Children						
1–3 y	300	15	15	6	30	0.5
4–8 y	400	25	15	7	55	0.6
Males						
9–13 y	600	45	15	11	60	0.9
14–18 y	900	75	15	15	75	1.2
19–30 y	900	90	15	15	120	1.2
31–50 y	900	90	15	15	120	1.2
51–70 y	900	90	15	15	120	1.2
>70 y	900	90	20	15	120	1.2
Females						
9–13 y	600	45	15	11	60	0.9
14–18 y	700	65	15	15	75	1.0
19–30 y	700	75	15	15	90	1.1
31–50 y	700	75	15	15	90	1.1
51–70 y	700	75	15	15	90	1.1
>70 y	700	75	20	15	90	1.1
Pregnancy						
14–18 y	750	80	15	15	75	1.4
19–30 y	770	85	15	15	90	1.4
31–50 y	770	85	15	15	90	1.4
Lactation						
14–18 y	1,200	115	15	19	75	1.4
19–30 y	1,300	120	15	19	90	1.4
31–50 y	1,300	120	15	19	90	1.4

RIBOFLAVIN (mg/d)	NIACIN (mg/d)	VIT B$_6$ (mg/d)	FOLATE (μ/d)	VITAMIN B$_{12}$ (μ/d)	PANTOTHENIC ACID (mg/d)	BIOTIN (μ/d)	CHOLINE (mg/d)
0.3	2	0.1	65	0.4	1.7	5	125
0.4	4	0.3	80	0.5	1.8	6	150
0.5	6	0.5	150	0.9	2	8	200
0.6	8	0.6	200	1.2	3	12	250
0.9	12	1.0	300	1.8	4	20	375
1.3	16	1.3	400	2.4	5	25	550
1.3	16	1.3	400	2.4	5	30	550
1.3	16	1.3	400	2.4	5	30	550
1.3	16	1.7	400	2.4	5	30	550
1.3	16	1.7	400	2.4	5	30	550
0.9	12	1.0	300	1.8	4	20	375
1.0	14	1.2	400	2.4	5	25	400
1.1	14	1.3	400	2.4	5	30	425
1.1	14	1.3	400	2.4	5	30	425
1.1	14	1.5	400	2.4	5	30	425
1.1	14	1.5	400	2.4	5	30	425
1.4	18	1.9	600	2.6	6	30	450
1.4	18	1.9	600	2.6	6	30	450
1.4	18	1.9	600	2.6	6	30	450
1.6	17	2.0	500	2.8	7	35	550
1.6	17	2.0	500	2.8	7	35	550
1.6	17	2.0	500	2.8	7	35	550

Mineral Micronutrients

LIFE STAGE GROUP	CALCIUM (mg/d)	CHROMIUM (μ/d)	COPPER (μ/d)	FLUORIDE (mg/d)	IODINE (μ/d)	IRON (mg/d)	MAGNESIUM (mg/d)
Infants							
0–6 mo	200	0.2	200	0.01	110	0.27	30
7–12 mo	260	5.5	220	0.5	130	11	75
Children							
1–3 y	700	11	340	0.7	90	7	80
4–8 y	1,000	15	440	1	90	10	130
Males							
9–13 y	1,300	25	700	2	120	8	240
14–18 y	1,300	35	890	3	150	11	410
19–30 y	1,000	35	900	4	150	8	400
31–50 y	1,000	35	900	4	150	8	420
51–70 y	1,000	30	900	4	150	8	420
>70 y	1,200	30	900	4	150	8	420
Females							
9–13 y	1,300	21	700	2	120	8	240
14–18 y	1,300	24	890	3	150	15	360
19–30 y	1,000	25	900	3	150	18	310
31–50 y	1,000	25	900	3	150	18	320
51–70 y	1,200	20	900	3	150	8	320
>70 y	1,200	20	900	3	150	8	320
Pregnancy							
14–18 y	1,300	29	1,000	3	220	27	400
19–30 y	1,000	30	1,000	3	220	27	350
31–50 y	1,000	30	1,000	3	220	27	360
Lactation							
14–18 y	1,300	44	1,300	3	290	10	360
19–30 y	1,000	45	1,300	3	290	9	310
31–50 y	1,000	45	1,300	3	290	9	320

MANGANESE (mg/d)	MOLYBDENUM (μ/d)	PHOSPHORUS (mg/d)	SELENIUM (μ/d)	ZINC (mg/d)	POTASSIUM (g/d)	SODIUM (g/d)	CHLORIDE (g/d)
0.003	2	100	15	2	0.4	0.12	0.18
0.6	3	275	20	3	0.7	0.37	0.57
1.2	17	460	20	3	3.0	1.0	1.5
1.5	22	500	30	5	3.8	1.2	1.9
1.9	34	1,250	40	8	4.5	1.5	2.3
2.2	43	1,250	55	11	4.7	1.5	2.3
2.3	45	700	55	11	4.7	1.5	2.3
2.3	45	700	55	11	4.7	1.5	2.3
2.3	45	700	55	11	4.7	1.3	2.0
2.3	45	700	55	11	4.7	1.2	1.8
1.6	34	1,250	40	8	4.5	1.5	2.3
1.6	43	1,250	55	9	4.7	1.5	2.3
1.8	45	700	55	8	4.7	1.5	2.3
1.8	45	700	55	8	4.7	1.5	2.3
1.8	45	700	55	8	4.7	1.3	2.0
1.8	45	700	55	8	4.7	1.2	1.8
2.0	50	1,250	60	12	4.7	1.5	2.3
2.0	50	700	60	11	4.7	1.5	2.3
2.0	50	700	60	11	4.7	1.5	2.3
2.6	50	1,250	70	13	5.1	1.5	2.3
2.6	50	700	70	12	5.1	1.5	2.3
2.6	50	700	70	12	5.1	1.5	2.3

APPENDIX C

Food as Medicine: Nutrient Index

NUTRIENT	SOURCE	NATURALLY OCCURRING FOODS
Proteins	Animal + plant	Dairy, fish, legumes, meat, nuts, poultry, shellfish, soy
Fats	Animal + plant	Dairy, fruits, fish, nuts, seeds, shellfish, soy, vegetables, vegetable oil
Carbohydrates	Animal + plant	Beans, dairy, fruits, legumes, sugar, vegetables, whole grains
VITAMINS		
Vitamin A	Animal + plant	Beef liver, butter, butternut squash, carrots, chicken livers, cod liver oil, cow's milk, eggs, kale, mustard greens, pumpkin, spinach, sweet potatoes
Thiamin	Mostly plant	Black beans, brown rice, cantaloupe, green peas, lentils, navy beans, oranges, pecans, pork, spinach, sunflower seeds, white rice, whole wheat bread
Riboflavin	Animal + plant	Almonds, beef, beet greens, chicken, cow dairy, eggs, soybeans, spinach, tempeh
Niacin	Animal + plant	Beef, chicken, cremini mushrooms, lamb, lentils, peanuts, tuna, turkey, salmon, whole wheat bread
Pantothenic acid	Animal + plant	Avocado, beef liver, chicken, cow dairy, lentils, lobster, shiitake mushrooms, sunflower seeds, sweet potatoes (skin on), trout
Vitamin B$_6$	Animal + plant	Avocado, bananas, beef, chicken, russet potatoes (skin on), spinach, sweet potatoes, tuna, turkey, wild salmon
Biotin	Animal + plant	Almonds, avocado, cauliflower, eggs, liver, oats, onions, peanuts, raspberries, salmon, sweet potatoes, tomatoes, whole wheat bread, yeast
Folate	Animal + plant	Asparagus, black beans, broccoli, chickpeas, kidney beans, lentils, lima beans, navy beans, orange juice, pinto beans, turnip greens, spinach

*Not a complete list.

NUTRIENT	SOURCE	NATURALLY OCCURRING FOODS
Vitamin B$_{12}$	Mostly animal	Beef, chicken, cod, cow dairy, clams, eggs, lamb, mackerel, miso, mussels, salmon, sardines, scallops, tempeh, tuna
Vitamin C	Plant	Broccoli, brussel sprouts, cantaloupe, cauliflower, grapefruits, kiwi, oranges, papaya, pineapple, potatoes, red bell peppers, spinach, strawberries
Vitamin D	Mostly animal	Eggs, cow dairy, mackerel, shiitake mushrooms, salmon, sardines, tuna
Vitamin E	Mostly plant	Almonds, apricots, avocados, beet greens, hazelnuts, mustard greens, peanuts, rainbow trout, spinach, sunflower seeds, swiss chard, turnip greens
Vitamin K	Mostly plant	Beet greens, broccoli, brussel sprouts, collard greens, green lettuce, kale, mustard greens, parsley, spinach, swiss chard, watercress
MINERALS		
Calcium	Animal + plant	Bok choy, broccoli, cheddar cheese, collard greens, cow dairy, kale, mustard greens, oranges, red beans, sardines, sesame seeds, spinach, tofu, white beans
Chromium	Animal + plant	Apples (with peel), bananas, barley, beef, broccoli, grapes, green beans, oats, oranges, potatoes, tomatoes, turkey breast
Copper	Animal + plant	Almonds, beef liver, cashews, chocolate, crab, hazelnuts, lentils, oysters, sesame seeds, shiitake mushrooms, soybeans, sunflower seeds, tempeh, walnuts
Iodine	Animal + plant	Cod, cow dairy, eggs, navy beans, potatoes (skin on), sardines, scallops, sea vegetables, shrimp, turkey, tuna
Iron	Animal + plant	Beef, chicken liver, chickpeas, kidney beans, lentils, mussels, navy beans, olives, oysters, quinoa, sesame seeds, soybeans, spinach, swiss chard, tofu, white beans
Magnesium	Animal + plant	Almonds, bananas, beet greens, blackstrap molasses, brown rice, cashews, cow dairy, hazelnuts, lima beans, mackerel, peanuts, pumpkin seeds, quinoa, soybeans, spinach, swiss chard

NUTRIENT	SOURCE	NATURALLY OCCURRING FOODS
MINERALS (continued)		
Manganese	Plant	Almonds, brown rice, chickpeas, green tea, oats, pecans, pineapple, pumpkin seeds, rye, soybeans, spinach, tempeh, whole wheat bread
Molybdenum	Mostly plant	Black beans, barley, chickpeas, kidney beans, green peas, lentils, lima beans, oats, pinto beans, soybeans
Phosphorus	Animal + plant	Almonds, chicken, cod, cow dairy, eggs, halibut, lentils, peanuts, pumpkin seeds, salmon, sardines, scallops, shrimp, soybeans, tempeh, tuna, turkey
Potassium	Mostly plant	Acorn squash, almonds, bananas, beet greens, beets, blackstrap molasses, bok choy, brussel sprouts, lima beans, oranges, prunes, potatoes (skin on), raisins, spinach, sweet potatoes, swiss chard, tuna
Selenium	Animal + plant	Beef, Brazil nuts, brown rice, chicken, clams, cod, halibut, lamb, oysters, salmon, sardines, scallops, shrimp, sunflower seeds, tuna, turkey
Sodium	—	Processed and salted foods
Zinc	Animal + plant	Almonds, beef, cashews, chickpeas, cow dairy, crab, lamb, lentils, oysters, pork, pumpkin seeds, quinoa, sesame seeds, shrimp, turkey

Source: The Linus Pauling Institute: Micronutrient Information Center and The World's Healthiest Foods

BIBLIOGRAPHY

Introduction

Eames-Sheavly, Marcia, Christine Hadekel, Angela M. Hedstrom, Amie Patchen, Robyn Stewart, and Jennifer Wilkins. "Discovering Our Food System." Ithaca, NY: Cornell University Cooperative Extension, 2011. https://cpb-us-e1.wpmucdn.com/blogs.cornell.edu/dist/f/575/files/2016/03/newlogoDiscovering-Our-Food-System-2lyk76c.pdf.

Nguyen, Binh T., and Lisa M. Powell. "The Impact of Restaurant Consumption among US Adults: Effects on Energy and Nutrient Intakes." *Public Health Nutrition* 17, no. 11 (November 2014): 2445–52. doi.org/10.1017/S1368980014001153.

Trubek, Amy B., Maria Carabello, Caitlin Morgan, and Jacob Lahne. "Empowered to Cook: The Crucial Role of 'Food Agency' in Making Meals." *Appetite* 116 (September 1, 2017): 297–305. doi.org/10.1016/j.appet.2017.05.017.

Utter, Jennifer, Nicole Larson, Melissa N. Laska, Megan Winkler, and Dianne Neumark-Sztainer. "Self-Perceived Cooking Skills in Emerging Adulthood Predict Better Dietary Behaviors and Intake 10 Years Later: A Longitudinal Study." *Journal of Nutrition Education and Behavior* 50, no. 5 (May 2018): 494–500. doi.org/10.1016/j.jneb.2018.01.021.

Chapter One

American Society for the Prevention of Cruelty to Animals. "Consumer Resources." www.aspca.org/shopwithyourheart/consumer-resources.

Arcury, Thomas A., Joseph G. Grzywacz, Dana B. Barr, Janeth Tapia, Haiying Chen, and Sara A. Quandt. "Pesticide Urinary Metabolite Levels of Children in Eastern North Carolina Farmworker Households." *Environmental Health Perspectives* 115, no. 8 (August 1, 2007): 1254–60. doi.org/10.1289/ehp.9975.

Baranski, Marcin, Dominika Srednicka-Tober, Nikolaos Volakakis, and Chris Seal. "Higher Antioxidant and Lower Cadmium Concentrations and Lower Incidence of Pesticide Residues in Organically Grown Crops: A Systematic Literature Review and Meta-analyses." *British Journal of Nutrition* 112, no. 5 (September 14, 2014): 794–811. doi.org/10.1017/S0007114514001366.

Bittman, Mark, and David L. Katz. "The Last Conversation You'll Ever Need to Have About Eating Right." *Grub Street*, 2018. www.grubstreet.com/2018/03/ultimate-conversation-on-healthy-eating-and-nutrition.html.

Black, Robert E. "Zinc Deficiency, Infectious Disease and Mortality in the Developing World." *The Journal of Nutrition* 133, no. 5 (May 2003): 1485S–89S. doi.org/10.1093/jn/133.5.1485S.

Borochov-Neori, Hamutal, Sylvie Judeinstein, Effi Tripler, Moti Harari, Ammon Greenberg, Ilan Shomer, and Doron Holland. "Seasonal and Cultivar Variations in Antioxidant and Sensory Quality of Pomegranate (*Punica ranatum L.*) Fruit." *Journal of Food Composition and Analysis* 22, no. 3 (May 2009): 189–95. doi.org/10.1016/j.jfca.2008.10.011.

Brantsaeter, Anne L., Trond A. Ydersbond, Jane A. Hoppin, Margaretha Haugen, and Helle M. Meltzer. "Organic Food in the Diet: Exposure and Health Implications." *Annual Review of Public Health* 38 (December 15, 2016): 295–313. doi.org/10.1146/annurev-publhealth-031816-044437.

Bruce D. G., D. J. Chisholm, L. H. Storlien, E. W. Kraegen, and G. A. Smythe. "The Effects of Sympathetic Nervous System Activation and Psychological Stress on Glucose Metabolism and Blood Pressure in Subjects with Type 2 (Non-insulin Dependent) Diabetes Mellitus." *Diabetologia* 35, no. 9 (September 1992): 835–43.

Ciancaleoni, Simona, Andrea Onofri, Renzo Torricelli, and Valeria Negri. "Broccoli Yield Response to Environmental Factors in Sustainable Agriculture." *European Journal of Agronomy* 72 (January 2016): 1–9. doi.org/10.1016/j.eja.2015.09.009.

Environmental Working Group. "Meat Eater's Guide to Climate Change + Health." http://static.ewg.org/reports/2011/meateaters/pdf/methodology_ewg_meat_eaters_guide_to_health_and_climate_2011.pdf.

Gancheva, Sofiya, and Michael Roden. "Central Regulation of Glucose Metabolism in Humans: Fact or Fiction?." *Diabetes* 65, no. 9 (September 2016): 2367–469. doi.org/10.2337/dbi16-0032.

George Mateljan Foundation. "Beef, Grass-fed." *The World's Healthiest Foods.* www.whfoods.com/genpage.php?tname=foodspice&dbid=141.

———. "Soybeans." *The World's Healthiest Foods.* www.whfoods.com/genpage.php?tname=foodspice&dbid=79.

———. "What Is Your Approach to Genetically Modified Foods?" *The World's Healthiest Foods.* www.whfoods.com/genpage.php?tname=george&dbid=428.

Greene, Catherine, Carolyn Dimitri, Biing-Hwan Lin, William D. Mcbride, Lydia Oberholtzer, and Travis A. Smith. "Emerging Issues in the U.S. Organic Industry." United States Department of Agriculture Economic Information Bulletin No. EIB-55, June 2009. www.ers.usda.gov/publications/pub-details/?pubid=44416.

Hingle, Melanie D., Jayanthi Kandiah, and Annette Maggi. "Practice Paper of the Academy of Nutrition and Dietetics: Selecting Nutrient-Dense Foods for Good Health." *Journal of the Academy of Nutrition and Dietetics* 116, no. 9 (September 2016): 1473–79. doi.org/10.1016/j.jand.2016.06.375.

Huen, Karen, Kim Harley, Jordan Brooks, Alan Hubbard, Asa Bradman, Brenda Eskenazi, and Nina Holland. "Developmental Changes in PON1 Enzyme Activity in Young Children and Effects of PON1 Polymorphisms." *Environmental Health Perspectives* 117, no. 10 (October 1, 2009): 1632–38. doi.org/10.1289/ehp.0900870.

Key, Nigel. "Farms that Sell Directly to Consumers May Stay in Business Longer." U.S. Department of Agriculture, April 28, 2016. www.usda.gov/media/blog/2016/04/28/farms-sell-directly-consumers-may-stay-business-longer.

Kim, Sang-Ha, Hyun-Mi Kim, Young-Min Ye, Seung-Hyun Kim, Dong-Ho Nahm, Hae-Sim Park, Sang-Ryeol Ryu, and Bou-Oung Lee. "Evaluating the Allergic Risk of Genetically Modified Soybean." *Yonsei Medical Journal* 47, no. 4 (August 2006): 505–12. doi.org/10.3349/ymj.2006.47.4.505.

Mahan, L. Kathleen, Sylvia Escott-Stump, and Janice L. Raymond. *Krause's Food and the Nutrition Care Process.* Thirteenth edition. St. Louis, MO: Elsevier Inc., 2012.

McAfee, A. J., E. M. McSorley, G. J. Cuskelly, and A. M. Fearon. "Red Meat from Animals Offered a Grass Diet Increases Plasma and Platelet *n*-3 PUFA in Healthy Consumers." *British Journal of Nutrition* 105, no. 1 (January 14, 2011): 80–89. doi.org/10.1017/S0007114510003090.

Mead, M. Nathaniel. "Nutrigenomics: The Genome-Food Interface." *Environmental Health Perspectives* 115, no. 12 (December 2007): 582–89. https://ehp.niehs.nih.gov/doi/10.1289/ehp.115-a582.

Melina, Vesanto, Winston Craig, and Susan Levin. "Position of the Academy of Nutrition and Dietetics: Vegetarian Diets." *Journal of the Academy of Nutrition and Dietetics* 116, no. 12 (December 2016): 1970–80. doi.org/10.1016/j.jand.2016.09.025.

Monday Campaigns. "Meatless Monday." www.meatlessmonday.com.

Pope, Victoria. "The Joy of Food." *National Geographic Magazine.* https://www.nationalgeographic.com/foodfeatures/joy-of-food.

Procter, Sandra B., and Christina G. Campbell. "Position of the Academy of Nutrition and Dietetics: Nutrition and Lifestyle for a Healthy Pregnancy Outcome." *Journal of the Academy of Nutrition and Dietetics* 114, no. 7 (July 2014): 1099–103. doi.org/10.1016/j.jand.2014.05.005.

Samsel, Anthony, and Stephanie Seneff. "Glyphosate, Pathways to Modern Diseases II: Celiac Sprue and Gluten Intolerance." *Interdisciplinary Toxicology* 6, no. 4 (December 2014): 159–84. doi.org/10.2478/intox-2013-0026.

Srednicka-Tober, Dominika, Marcin Baranski, Chris Seal, and Roy Sanderson. "Higher PUFA and n-3 PUFA, Conjugated Linoleic Acid, α-Tocopherol and Iron, but Lower Iodine and Selenium Concentrations in Organic Milk: A Systematic Literature Review and Meta- and Redundancy Analyses." *British Journal of Nutrition* 115, no. 6 (March 28, 2016): 1043–60. doi.org/10.1017/S0007114516000349.

Timmerman, Gayle M., and Adama Brown. "The Effect of a Mindful Restaurant Eating Intervention on Weight Management in Women." *Journal of Nutrition Education and Behavior* 44, no. 1 (January–February 2012): 22–28. doi.org/10.1016/j.jneb.2011.03.143.

Tribole, Evelyn, and Elyse Resch. *Intuitive Eating: A Revolutionary Program That Works.* New York: St. Martin's Press, 2012.

Trubek, Amy B., Maria Carabello, Caitlin Morgan, and Jacob Lahne. "Empowered to Cook: The Crucial Role of 'Food Agency' in Making Meals." *Appetite* 116 (September 1, 2017): 297–305. doi.org/10.1016/j.appet.2017.05.017.

U.S. Department of Agriculture. "Organic Labeling Standards." www.ams.usda.gov/grades-standards/organic-labeling-standards.

———. "Organic Production & Handling Standards." November 2016. www.ams.usda.gov/publications/content/organic-production-handling-standards.

———. "Soybeans & Oil Crops." Last updated August 29, 2019. www.ers.usda.gov/topics/crops/soybeans-oil-crops.

———. "Wheat: Data & Analysis." www.fas.usda.gov/commodities/wheat.

U.S. Department of Health and Human Services and U.S. Department of Agriculture. *2015–2020 Dietary Guidelines for Americans*, 8th ed. December 2015. https://health.gov/dietaryguidelines/2015/resources/2015-2020_Dietary_Guidelines.pdf.

U.S. Environmental Protection Agency. "Pesticides and Food: Healthy, Sensible Food Practices." www.epa.gov/safepestcontrol/pesticides-and-food-healthy-sensible-food-practices.

U.S. Food & Drug Administration. "Non-TDS Foods Analyzed for PCDD/PCDFs." Last updated April 22, 2019. https://wayback.archive-it.org/7993/20190422162650/https://www.fda.gov/Food/FoodborneIllnessContaminants/ChemicalContaminants/ucm2006782.htm.

VanEpps, Eric M., and Christina A. Roberto. "The Influence of Sugar-Sweetened Beverage Warnings." *American Journal of Preventative Medicine* 51, no. 5 (November 2016): 664–72. doi.org/10.1016/j.amepre.2016.07.010.

Vedantam, Shankar. "Why Eating the Same Food Increases People's Trust and Cooperation." Interview by David Greene. *Hidden Brain*, NPR, February 2, 2017. Audio 3:26. https://www.npr.org/2017/02/02/512998465/why-eating-the -same-food-increases-peoples-trust-and-cooperation.

Winkens, Laura H. H., Tatjana van Strien, Juan R. Barrada, Ingeborg A. Brouwer, Brenda W. J. H. Penninx, and Marjolein Visser. "The Mindful Eating Behavior Scale: Developmental and Psychometric Properties in a Sample of Dutch Adults Aged 55 Years and Older." *Journal of the Academy of Nutrition and Dietetics* 118, no. 7 (July 2018): 1277–90. doi.org/10.1016/j.jand.2018.01.015.

Wolfram, Taylor. "Processed Foods: What's OK and What to Avoid." February 11, 2019. www.eatright.org/food/nutrition/nutrition-facts-and-food-labels /processed-foods-whats-ok-and-what-to-avoid.

Wood, Rebecca. *The New Whole Foods Encyclopedia*. New York: Penguin Group, 2010.

Chapter 2

Brown-Riggs, Constance. "Functional Fibers—Research Shows They Provide Health Benefits Similar to Intact Fibers in Whole Foods." *Today's Dietitian* 15, no. 12 (December 2013): 32. www.todaysdietitian.com/newarchives/120913p32.shtml.

Center for Ecogenetics and Environmental Health, University of Washington. "Fast Facts About The Human Microbiome." January 2014. https://depts.washington.edu /ceeh/downloads/FF_Microbiome.pdf.

George Mateljan Foundation. "Sea Vegetables." *The World's Healthiest Foods*. www.whfoods.com/genpage.php?tname=foodspice&dbid=135.

Greenstein Luna. "Mental Health Is a Balancing Act." National Alliance on Mental Illness. March 17, 2017. www.nami.org/blogs/nami-blog/march-2017/mental -health-is-a-balancing-act.

Guiry, Michael D. "Seaweed as Human Food." *The Seaweed Site*. www.seaweed.ie /uses_general/humanfood.php.

Harvard Health Publishing. "Nutrition's Dynamic Duos." *Harvard Health Letter*. July 2009. www.health.harvard.edu/newsletter_article/Nutritions-dynamic-duos.

———. "The Truth about Fats: The Good, the Bad, and the In-between." Last updated August 18, 2018. www.health.harvard.edu/staying-healthy/the-truth-about -fats-bad-and-good.

Jacobs, David R., and Linda C. Tapsell. "Food Synergy: The Key to a Healthy Diet." *Proceedings of the Nutrition Society* 72, no. 2 (May 2013): 200–206. doi.org/10.1017 /S0029665112003011.

Katz, Sandor. *The Art of Fermentation: An In-Depth Exploration of Essential Concepts and Processes from Around the World*. Vermont: Chelsea Green Publishing, 2012.

Linus Pauling Institute. "Micronutrient Information Center." Oregon State University. https://lpi.oregonstate.edu/mic.

Manz, F. "Hydration and Disease." *Journal of the American College of Nutrition* 26, no. 5 (October 2007 supplement): 535S–41S. www.tandfonline.com/doi/abs/10.1080/07315724.2007.10719655.

Margulis, Lynn, and Dorion Sagan. *Microcosmos: Four Billion Years of Evolution from Our Microbial Ancestors*. New York: Summit Books, 1986.

Merriam-Webster. "Health." www.merriam-webster.com/dictionary/health.

National Academies of Sciences, Engineering, and Medicine. "Dietary Reference Intakes: Macronutrients." www.nationalacademies.org/hmd/~/media/Files/Activity%20Files/Nutrition/DRI-Tables/8_Macronutrient%20Summary.pdf?la=en.

Popkin, Barry M., Kristen E. D'Anci, and Irwin H. Rosenberg. "Water, Hydration, and Health." *Nutrition Reviews* 68, no. 8 (August 1, 2010): 439–58. doi.org/10.1111/j.1753-4887.2010.00304.x.

Prasad, Sahdeo, and Bharat B. Aggarwal. "Turmeric, the Golden Spice." In *Herbal Medicine: Biomolecular and Clinical Aspects*, ed. F. F. Benzie and Sissi Wachtel-Galor, Chapter 13. Boca Raton, FL: CRC Press, 2011.

Reed, Stacy, and Nancy Wiker. "Physical Activity for Best Bone Health." PennState Extension, College of Agricultural Sciences. Last updated August 14, 2014. https://extension.psu.edu/physical-activity-for-best-bone-health.

Schaeffer, Juliann. "Color Me Healthy—Eating for a Rainbow of Benefits." *Today's Dietitian* 10, no. 11 (November 2008): 32. www.todaysdietitian.com/newarchives/110308p34.shtml.

Schulzova, V., J. Hajslova, R. Peroutka, J. Gry, and H. C. Andersson. "Influence of Storage and Household Processing on the Agaritine Content of the Cultivated *Agaricus* Mushroom." *Food Additives and Contaminants* 19, no. 9 (September 2002): 853–62.

Seely, Dugald, and Rana Singh. "Adaptogenic Potential of a Polyherbal Natural Health Product: Report on a Longitudinal Clinical Trial." *Evidence-Based Complementary and Alternative Medicine* 4, no. 3 (September 2007): 375–80. dx.doi.org/10.1093/ecam/nel101.

Shreiner, Andrew B., John Y. Kao, and Vincent B. Young. "The Gut Microbiome in Health and in Disease." *Current Opinion in Gastroenterology* 31, no. 1 (January 2015): 69–75. https://insights.ovid.com/pubmed?pmid=25394236.

Stamets, Paul. "Place Mushrooms in Sunlight to Get Your Vitamin D: Part One." *Huffington Post*. Last updated December 7, 2017. www.huffpost.com/entry /mushrooms-vitamin-d_n_1635941.

Thalheimer, Judith. "The Top 5 Soy Myths." *Today's Dietitian* 16, no. 4 (April 2014): 52. www.todaysdietitian.com/newarchives/040114p52.shtml.

U.S. Department of Agriculture. "ChooseMyPlate." www.choosemyplate.gov.

U.S. Department of Health and Human Services. "Physical Activity Guidelines for Americans." https://health.gov/paguidelines/second-edition/pdf/physical_ activity_guidelines_2nd_edition.pdf.

Wilson, Michael. *Microbial Inhabitants of Humans: Their Ecology and Role in Health and Disease*. Cambridge, UK: Cambridge University Press, 2010.

Youdim, Adrienne. "Overview of Nutrition." *Merck Manual*. Last updated May 2019. www.merckmanuals.com/professional/nutritional-disorders /nutrition-general-considerations/overview-of-nutrition?qt=&sc=&alt.

Chapter 3

Goldsmith, Ellen, and Maya Klein. *Nutritional Healing with Chinese Medicine*. Toronto: Robert Rose, Inc., 2017.

Watson-Tara, Marlene. "The Five Tastes: Balancing Foods for All Seasons." T. Colin Campbell Center for Nutrition Studies. August 14, 2015. https://nutritionstudies .org/the-five-tastes-balancing-foods-for-all-seasons.

Zimecki, Michal. "The Lunar Cycle: Effects on Human and Animal Behavior and Physiology." *Advances in Hygiene and Experimental Medicine* 60 (January 2006): 1–7. http://www.phmd.pl/api/files/view/1953.pdf.

Chapter 4

Achitoff-Gray, Niki. "Cooking Fats 101: What's a Smoke Point and Why Does It Matter?" Serious Eats. Last updated September 25, 2019. www.seriouseats.com/2014/05 /cooking-fats-101-whats-a-smoke-point-and-why-does-it-matter.html.

America's Test Kitchen. "Flavoring Dried Beans with Seaweed." *Cook's Illustrated*. www.cooksillustrated.com/how_tos/6385-flavoring-dried-beans-with-seaweed.

Cleveland Clinical. "Health Essentials: What You Should Know About Beans and the (Embarrassing) Gas They Cause." September 20, 2018. https://health.cleveland clinic.org/the-musical-fruit-what-you-should-know-about-beans-and-gas/.

Delaware Sea Grant. "Seafood Handling and Storage." *Seafood Health Facts: Making Smart Choices*. 2019. www.seafoodhealthfacts.org/seafood-safety /general-information-patients-and-consumers/seafood-handling-and-storage.

Environmental Working Group. "Shopper's Guide to Pesticides in Produce." 2019. www.ewg.org/foodnews.

George Mateljan Foundation. "What Is the Best Way to Roast Nuts and Seeds?" *The World's Healthiest Foods*. www.whfoods.com/genpage php?tname= george&dbid=359.

Harvard Health Publishing. "Trending Now: Sprouted Grains." *Harvard Health Letter*. November 2017. www.health.harvard.edu/staying-healthy/trending-now -sprouted-grains.

Jang, Yu K., Mee Y. Lee, Hyang Y. Kim, Sarah Lee, Soo H. Yeo, Seong Y. Baek, and Choong H. Lee. "Comparison of Traditional and Commercial Vinegars Based on Metabolite Profiling and Antioxidant Activity." *Journal of Microbiology and Biotechnology* 25, no. 2 (February 2015): 217–26. dx.doi.org/10.4014/jmb.1408.08021.

Konieczna, Aleksandra, Aleksandra Rutkowska, and Dominik Rachon. "Health Risk of Exposure to Bisphenol A (BPA)." *Annals of the National Institute of Hygiene* 66, no. 1 (September 2015): 5–11. https://pdfs.semanticscholar.org/916c/a7faa290e73baa ae39c19d9f5c794c9781cb.pdf.

Lair, Cynthia. *Sourdough on the Rise*. Seattle: Sasquatch Books, 2019.

Monterey Bay Aquarium. "Helping People Make Better Seafood Choices for a Healthy Ocean." *Seafood Watch*. www.seafoodwatch.org.

Nestle, Marion. *What to Eat*. New York: North Point Press, 2007.

Newgent, Jackie. "How to Use Plastic Food Storage Containers." *Eat Right*. February 21, 2019. www.eatright.org/homefoodsafety/four-steps/refrigerate /how-to-use-plastic-food-storage-containers.

Nyombaire, G., M. Siddiq, and K. Dolan. "Effect of Soaking and Cooking on the Oli- gosaccharides and Lectins in Red Kidney Beans (Phaseolus Vulgaris L.)." Department of Food Science and Human Nutrition, Michigan State University. 2010. https://naldc.nal.usda.gov/download/IND43940829/PDF.

"Preserving the Nutrients of Food with Proper Care." *New York Times*, July 7, 1982. www.nytimes.com/1982/07/07/garden/preserving-the-nutrients-of-food-with -proper-care.html.

Ruhs, Barbara. "The Retail RD: Food Environments Designed to Sell." *Today's Dietitian* 19, no. 5 (May 2017)." https://www.todaysdietitian.com/newarchives/ 0517p20.shtml.

University of California–Davis, Produce for Better Health Foundation. "Storing Fresh Fruits and Vegetables for Best Flavor." 2012. www.fruitsandveggiesmore matters.org/wp-content/uploads/UserFiles/File/pdf/why/Storing_Fruits_Veggies _FINAL.pdf.

Utah State University Extension. "Food Storage: Dry Beans." https://extension.usu .edu/foodstorage/howdoi/dry_beans.

Weil, Andrew. "Are Plastic Containers Unhealthy?" *Weil*. November 2, 2006. www.drweil.com/health-wellness/balanced-living/healthy-living/are-plastic -containers-unhealthy/.

Wirden, Marc, Constance Delaugerre, Anne G. Marcelin, et al. "Comparison of the Dynamics of Resistance-Associated Mutations to Nucleoside Reverse Transcriptase Inhibitors, Nonnucleoside Reverse Transcriptase Inhibitors, and Protease Inhibitors after Cessation of Antiretroviral Combination Therapy." *Antimicrobial Agents and Chemotherapy* 48, no. 2 (February 2004): 644–47. doi.org/10.1128 /aac.48.2.644-647.2004.

Chapters 5–9

Mateljan, George. *The World's Healthiest Foods*. Seattle: George Mateljan Foundation, 2015.

Oldways Whole Grains Council. "Cooking with Whole Grains." https://wholegrains council.org/recipes/cooking-whole-grains.

Oregon State University. "Linus Pauling Institute: Micronutrient Information Center." https://lpi.oregonstate.edu/mic.

Oregon State University Extension. "Storing Food for Safety and Quality." https:// catalog.extension.oregonstate.edu/sites/catalog/files/project/pdf/pnw612.pdf

University of California–Davis. "Beans Cooking Chart." https://shcs.ucdavis.edu /sites/default/files/documents/BeansCookingChart.pdf.

U.S. Department of Health & Human Services. "Cold Food Storage Chart." https://www.foodsafety.gov/food-safety-charts/cold-food-storage-charts.

RESOURCES

Find a Registered Dietitian Nutritionist

Academy of Nutrition and Dietetics—Registered Dietitian Nutritionists
www.eatright.org/find-an-expert

Dietitians in Integrative and Functional Medicine—Integrative RD
https://integrativerd.org/find_an_rd

Institute of Functional Medicine Practitioners
www.ifm.org/find-a-practitioner

Integrative and Functional Nutrition Academy—Graduate Directory
www.ifnacademy.com/meet-the-experts/meet-our-grads

Intuitive Eating Counselor Directory
www.intuitiveeating.org/certified-counselors

Nutrition Information

Dietary Guidelines for Americans
health.gov/dietaryguidelines

Eat Right: The Academy of Nutrition and Dietetics
www.eatright.org

Linus Pauling Institute: Micronutrient Information Center
lpi.oregonstate.edu/mic

National Institutes of Health: Office of Dietary Supplements
ods.od.nih.gov/Health_Information/Dietary_Reference_Intakes.aspx

The World's Healthiest Foods—Nutrient database
  whfoods.org

USDA ChooseMyPlate
  www.choosemyplate.gov

Certified Food Labels

American Grassfed Association
  www.americangrassfed.org

Certified Humane
  certifiedhumane.org/wp-content/uploads/HFAC-Volunteer-Guide.pdf

Fair Trade Certified
  www.fairtradecertified.org

Non-GMO Project
  www.nongmoproject.org

USDA Organic
  www.usda.gov/topics/organic

Organic and Seasonal Produce

Environmental Working Group—Dirty Dozen and Clean Fifteen
  www.ewg.org/foodnews/dirty-dozen.php

USDA National Farmers Market Directory
  www.ams.usda.gov/local-food-directories/farmersmarkets

USDA SNAP-Ed Connection
  snaped.fns.usda.gov/seasonal-produce-guide

Sustainability

Eat Wild
  www.eatwild.com/products/index.html

Monterey Bay Aquarium Seafood Watch
  www.seafoodwatch.org

Slow Food USA
  http://slowfoodusa.org

INDEX

A

acai purée, 163
adaptogens, 50
aerobic activities, 56
aging, 32, 34, 35, 52
allspice, whole berries, 112
almond butter, 16
    Flourless Chocolate Almond Butter
        Brownies, 161–62
    Roasted Banana and Almond Butter
        Breakfast Cookies, 167
    Strawberry Vanilla Almond Butter
        Smoothie, 121
    Vanilla Tofu Frosting, 137
almond flour
    Roasted Banana and Almond Butter
        Breakfast Cookies, 167
    Strawberry Rhubarb Crisp, 139
almonds, 167
    Almond Milk, 99, 121
    Broccoli Salad, 169–70
    Dark Chocolate Banana Bread, 207
    Roasted Chicken Salad, 177
    Tangy Italian Cauliflower Salad, 171
American Cancer Society, 44
American Journal of Preventive Medicine, 17
amino acids, 32–33, 100, 127
animals, humane treatment of, 12–13, 74
anthocyanins, 41, 163, 191–93
antibiotics, 7, 12, 13
antioxidants
    mineral sources, 37, 38
    in rainbow foods, 39
    in sea vegetables, 48

    in spices and herbs, 50, 51, 103
    in vinegars, 90
    vitamin sources, 35, 36
anxiety, 22–23, 25, 28, 46, 55, 61, 62, 143
apples
    Cinnamon Apple Overnight Oats, 168
    Mini Whole Wheat Apple Galettes, 183–85
applesauce, 92, 137
arrowroot powder, 139
Art of Fermentation, The (Katz), 46
asparagus, 112, 125, 131
avocados, 39, 70, 188–89
    Egg Muffins, 144
    Simplest Tempeh Tacos, The, 155–57
    Spicy Sriracha Mung Bean Bowl, 127–29

B

baking ingredients, 90–91
balance, 31–32, 52–55, 56
bananas
    Dark Chocolate Banana Bread, 207
    freezing, 70
    Roasted Banana and Almond Butter
        Breakfast Cookies, 167
    Strawberry Vanilla Almond Butter
        Smoothie, 121
basil
    Basil Oil, 147
    Basil Walnut Pesto, 132
batch cooking, 69, 96, 116, 127–29, 188–89
beans, 69, 77
    black, Loaded Sweet Potatoes, 204
    cooking and soaking, 113–14
    organic, 11–12

244

mirin, 133–34, 178
miso, 44, 80
   Mirin and Miso Glazed Cod, 178
   Roasted Brussel Sprouts, 199
   Vegetable Miso Soup, 126
molasses, blackstrap, 91, 205–6
molybdenum, 38
Monterey Bay Seafood Watch Consumer Guide,
   75, 152
Morales, Bonnie, 181
muscle-strengthening activities, 56
mushrooms, 48, 50, 61, 84
   enoki, 126
   raw, 84
   shiitake, 133–34
   storing, 69, 84
mustard seeds, 107, 112

N

National Alliance on Mental Illness (NAMI), 56
nervous system
   carbohydrates and, 34
   parasympathetic, 23, 26
   support for, 35–36, 37, 197
   sympathetic, 22–23
neurological development and disorders, 33, 35,
   37, 46, 48
nut butters
   Cashew Butter Stuffed Dates, 209
   Ginger Almond Sauce, 153–54
   instructions, 108
   See also almond butter
nutmeg
   Carrot Cake Cupcakes, 137
   Chocolate and Chai Spiced Granola, 190
   Cinnamon Apple Overnight Oats, 168
   Mini Whole Wheat Apple Galettes, 183–85
   Strawberry Rhubarb Crisp, 139
nutrient density and diversity, 13, 16, 53, 83,
   190
nutrigenomics, 4
nutrition, xi
   assimilating, 23, 28
   conflicting information about, xiii
   individualized needs for, 31, 52
   of organic vs. conventional foods, 8–9, 12, 14
   supplementation, 38
nuts
   hazelnuts, 190
   organic vs. conventional, 14

pecans, 139, 190
pistachios, 39
storing, 69, 77–79
See also almonds; cashews; walnuts

O

oats, rolled
   Chocolate and Chai Spiced Granola, 190
   Cinnamon Apple Overnight Oats, 168
   Roasted Banana and Almond Butter
     Breakfast Cookies, 167
   Strawberry Rhubarb Crisp, 139
Oh She Glows blog (Liddon), 175
oils, 45
   avocado, 127–29, 144, 155–57
   refined, 17–19
   smoke points, 80, 101
   storing, 69, 79–80
   walnut, 137
   See also coconut oil; olive oil; sesame oil,
     toasted
olive oil
   Basil Oil, 147
   Basil Walnut Pesto, 132
   Chimichurri Corn, 152
   Garlic Vinaigrette, 195–96
   Quinoa Tabbouleh, 151
   smoke point, 80
   Tangy Italian Cauliflower Salad, 171
   Tarragon Vinaigrette, 131
olives
   black, 171
   Castelvetrano or green, 179
omega-3 fatty acids, 13
   benefits of, 33–34, 45
   in organic food, 9, 12
   sources of, 41, 44, 79, 131, 159–60, 182
onions
   red, 169–70, 171, 173, 177
   spring, 122
   See also onions, white or yellow; scallions;
     shallots
onions, white or yellow
   Beef and Beet Borscht, 181
   Bone Broth (Chicken), 100
   Coconut Curry Red Lentil Stew, 175–76
   Creamy Red Pepper and Tomato Soup, 147
   Egg Muffins, 144
   Loaded Sweet Potatoes, 204
   Simplest Tempeh Tacos, 155–57

soybeans, 44
    cooking and soaking, 113–14
    organic, 11–12
    Simplest Tempeh Tacos, 155–57
    See also miso; tofu
spices, 50–52, 69, 84–87
spinach, 83
    Coconut Curry Red Lentil Stew, 175–76
    Cultured Key Lime Cashew Yogurt, 143
spiritual health, xiii, 57
sprouts, growing, 117
squash, 39
    butternut, 173
    kabocha, 203
stocks
    beef, 181
    homemade, 67
    vegetable, 135, 175–76, 197
strawberries
    Infused Water, 105
    Strawberry Almond Milk, 99
    Strawberry Rhubarb Crisp, 139
    Strawberry Vanilla Almond Butter Smoothie,
        121
superfoods, 82, 83
supplementation, 38
sustainability
    food purchases supporting, 21–22
    health and, xii
    of organic farming, 7
    of sea vegetables, 82
    of seafood, 75
sweet potatoes, 204
sweeteners
    allergies and, 53
    brown sugar, 207
    coconut sugar, 139, 205–6
    maple sugar, 205–6
    refined, 17
    storing, 69, 91–92
    Sucanat, 139
    See also honey; maple syrup

T
tarragon, 131, 169–70
thyroid health, 37, 38, 44
tofu, 153
    Chocolate Tofu Mousse, 182
    Vanilla Tofu Frosting, 137

Vegetable Fried Brown Rice, 133–34
    Vegetable Miso Soup, 126
tomato paste, 147
tomato sauce, 197
tomatoes, 39, 41
    canned, 175–76, 197
    Creamy Red Pepper and Tomato Soup, 147
    Quinoa Tabbouleh, 151
turmeric, 50–51
    Coconut Curry Red Lentil Stew, 175–76
    Curried Cauliflower (fermented), 107
    Golden Turmeric Paste, 103, 203
Turshen, Julia, 132
Twenty-Minute Challenge, 23

V
vanilla beans/vanilla bean paste
    Vanilla Tofu Frosting, 137
    Vegetable Fried Brown Rice, 133–34
    Vegetable Miso Soup, 126
vanilla extract, 90, 207
    in beverages, 99, 121
    in breakfast foods, 145–46, 167, 168, 188,
        190
    in desserts, 137, 139, 161–62, 182
vegetables, 41–43
    cruciferous, increasing nutrients in, 123
    organic, 9–11
    seasons and, 61
    storing, 72
    washing, 11
vinegars
    apple cider, 100, 112, 173
    red wine, 127–29, 152
    sherry, 131
    storing, 69, 90
    white wine, 127–29, 171, 179
    See also rice wine vinegar
vitamin C, 19, 36
    iron and, 3, 37
    sources of, 39, 41, 48, 125, 151, 169–70, 171,
        199
vitamins, 34–35
    fat- or water-soluble, 34, 45
    vitamin A, x–xi, 35, 125, 151
    vitamin D, 36, 37, 48, 159–60
    vitamin E, 43, 131
    vitamin K, 41, 43, 151, 169–70, 199
    See also vitamin C; vitamins, B

vitamins, B, 35–36
    B2 (riboflavin), 122
    B6 (pyridoxine), 122
    B12 (cobalamin), 28, 159–60, 178
    fermented foods and, 45
    sources of, 43, 48, 72, 157, 173
    See also biotin; folate

W

walnuts
    Basil Walnut Pesto, 132
    Chocolate and Chai Spiced Granola, 190
    Cinnamon Apple Overnight Oats, 168
    Roasted Banana and Almond Butter Breakfast
        Cookies, 167
    Strawberry Rhubarb Crisp, 139
water, 34, 52, 105
Waters, Alice, 58
weight, x
    body movement and, 55
    body rhythms and, 60
    mindful eating and, 25
    obesity, 3, 17–18, 33, 43, 60
    seasons and, 61
whole foods, 5, 19, 38, 83. *See also* nutrient
    density and diversity
whole grains, 14–16, 17, 43, 54, 64, 72–73,
    115–16

whole wheat flour
    Dark Chocolate Banana Bread, 207
    Homemade Whole Wheat Toaster Waffles,
        188–89
    Whole Wheat and Flax Tortillas, 157
whole wheat pastry flour
    Carrot Cake Cupcakes, 137
    Mini Whole Wheat Apple Galettes, 183–85
    Spiced Whole Wheat Ginger and Molasses
        Cookies, 205–6
WWGD (What Would Grandma Do)?, 6

Y

yeast, 188–89
yogurt, 45
    Beef and Beet Borscht, 181
    Cinnamon Apple Overnight Oats, 168
    Cultured Key Lime Cashew Yogurt, 143
    Herb Yogurt Dressing, 169–70
    Loaded Sweet Potatoes, 204
    Plain Whole Milk Yogurt, 110–11
    Poppy Seed Yogurt Dressing, 177
    Spicy Sriracha Mung Bean Bowl, 127–29
    Spicy Three Bean Chili, 181, 197

Z

zinc, 14, 39, 43
zucchini, 41, 159–60

ABOUT THE AUTHOR

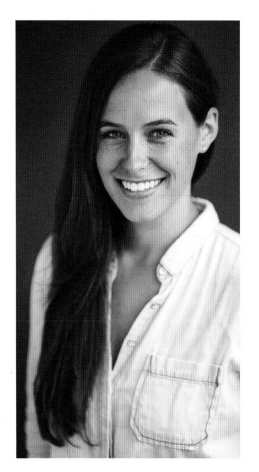

Carly Knowles, MS, RDN, LD, has always loved cooking, but it wasn't until she lived in a rural village in Peru that she saw just how impactful food and nutrition can be. It was a profound moment that made her realize that food truly is medicine and set her on a path to becoming a Registered Dietitian Nutritionist (RDN) and food and nutrition expert. She earned her Master of Science degree in nutrition from Bastyr University and has experience working as a clinical dietitian in both inpatient and outpatient settings as well as private practice. Carly now teaches cooking classes in the community and specializes in food and nutrition writing, recipe development, and nutrition consulting for healthy food and cookware brands. On her website (CarlyKnowles.com), you can find inspired, flavorful recipes that focus on whole foods to nourish good health and bring joy. This is her first book. Carly lives in the Pacific Northwest with her husband and son.